# EMBRACING DEMENTIA

# EMBRACING DEMENTIA

## Real-Life Experiences of Providing Optimal Dementia Care

Melissa Johnson,
RN, MHA, CHPN, CCM

JONES MEDIA
PUBLISHING

Jones Media Publishing
10645 N. Tatum Blvd. Ste. 200-166
Phoenix, AZ 85028
www.JonesMediaPublishing.com

Disclaimer:

The author strives to be as accurate and complete as possible in the creation of this book, notwithstanding the fact that the author does not warrant or represent at any time that the contents within are accurate due to the rapidly changing nature of the Internet.

While all attempts have been made to verify information provided in this publication, the Author and the Publisher assume no responsibility and are not liable for errors, omissions, or contrary interpretation of the subject matter herein. The Author and Publisher hereby disclaim any liability, loss, or damage incurred as a result of the application and utilization, whether directly or indirectly, of any information, suggestion, advice, or procedure in this book. Any perceived slights of specific persons, peoples, or organizations are unintentional.

In practical advice books, like anything else in life, there are no guarantees of income made. Readers are cautioned to rely on their own judgment about their individual circumstances to act accordingly. Readers are responsible for their own actions, choices, and results. This book is not intended for use as a source of legal, business, accounting, or financial advice. All readers are advised to seek the services of competent professionals in legal, business, accounting, and finance field.

Printed in the United States of America

ISBN: 978-1-948382-22-9 paperback
JMP2021.7

For those impacted by dementia . . .
may we find the strength to persevere.

# CONTENTS

# AUTHOR'S PREFACE

If you are a caregiver, medical professional, or a family member of a person with dementia, this book is for you. I congratulate your efforts in pursuing information to broaden your understanding of dementia. I hope this book equips you with tools needed along this journey, provides insight into topics that are not talked about often enough, and gives you the strength in knowing you are not alone.

This book will guide you through providing optimal care to a person with dementia, from diagnosis until the end of life. The narratives in this book are based on real-life experiences in my role as a Care Manager and Dementia Educator. Names and discernable information have been changed to protect the identity of those I have cared for, without removing the indispensable facts that make these stories intriguing, relatable, and teachable. Chapters are formatted in two distinct methods: Some chapters focus on real life scenarios interlaced with educational information. Other chapters focus on educational information interlaced with examples based on real-life encounters. This method is intended to provide extensive information in a relatable fashion to help guide you through how to cope and manage challenging times, while finding the beauty in the special moments. I also provide a variety of resources throughout the book. At the conclusion of this book, I have included a resource list.

After completing nursing school, I worked in an intensive care unit (ICU) in a hospital that mostly served the elderly. The interactions I generally had were with machines and rarely with patients. Nursing school provided a wealth of information; however, I felt ill-equipped in dementia care. Even though there were interactions with persons with dementia during clinicals, I found myself more curious about dementia coming out of nursing school. As a new nurse, I was scared in a way that made me meticulous and yearning to learn more.

At the beginning of shifts, nurses would pick their assignment for the night. For one of my memorable shifts, nurses seemed to avoid Doris, so I picked her. Doris, who was in her eighties, was being closely monitored after a confirmed case of urosepsis (sepsis from an infection in the urinary tract). Doris also had a diagnosis of dementia. She was not on a ventilator and was getting just a few medications through intravenous (IV) access. The other nurses passed her up as part of their assignment, which I found strange because she seemed much less complex than a patient with a ventilator, multiple IVs, and complex medical issues. Doris seemed very sweet and pleasant. She was cooperative during my assessment and took her medications when I asked. As the night went on, Doris started to exhibit behaviors which allowed me to have the first of many personal lessons on dementia. Doris pulled her IV out and got out of bed, causing alarms to ring loudly. I went to check on her and was able to get her to lie back down. The alarms went off again and she was out of the bed and naked. She was very agitated and disoriented. Her agitation continued to increase and her fear from disorientation persisted. She eventually received medication to help with agitation, then she finally calmed down. I was told, after the fact, infections in persons with dementia can cause behaviors, which is why the other nurses preferred a ventilator patient. This was the beginning of a career in caring for the elderly and working with many people with dementia and assisting their loved ones.

While an ICU nurse, I had an incredible experience with a gentleman and his wife and daughter. He had end-stage chronic obstructive pulmonary disease (COPD) and was declining despite all efforts. I spent time with him and his family talking about hospice, which they decided was the best option. He remained in the ICU for several hours until hospice could transport him to an inpatient unit. While waiting for transport I provided comfort care, which was different than the lifesaving care I was used to. The gentleman died a few days later. His wife and daughter came to the ICU with cookies and a card for me. The daughter hugged me and handed me a card. She whispered in my ear, "You were my dad's guardian angel." Inside the thoughtfully written card was an angel pin. I was so touched by this experience that I decided hospice is where I belonged

I spent the next five years in various aspects of hospice, such as case management, charge nurse in the inpatient unit, and eventually, management. There were many patients on hospice with end-stage dementia, and I was always drawn to them. I have admittedly been kicked, hit, spit on, screamed at, and had objects thrown at me. The more I learned, the more intrigued I was. I saw a greater need in my community, and after learning about geriatric care management, I decided, with the help of my husband, to start a care management business, using my skills in a much more meaningful way. I was called into complex situations when care was not managed optimally, and families were not sure where to turn. Generally, family members lived far away and needed an advocate for their loved one, and generally my clients had cognitive impairment. I took my clients to doctor's appointments, assisted in managing their medications, provided education and guidance to family members, went to the hospital when a client was sent, and continued in my role until the end of life.

I am often asked if difficulty with memory means dementia is present. The answer is no. There is some element of the aging process that contributes to deficits in memory, and as you can imagine, the older brain does not work the same as a forty-year-old brain. As a person ages, they may be slower, have more difficulty juggling multiple tasks, or make occasional mistakes. With dementia, a person will have difficulty concentrating, have poor judgment, have trouble managing money, and get confused when planning or thinking. As a people age, they may have difficulty thinking of a word, lose their train of thought when speaking, or require more concentration to keep up with a conversation. With dementia, people will have frequent issues finding words, regularly lose their train of thought, and have trouble conversating with others. As a person ages, they may forget the exact date but are able to figure it out, or they may walk into a room and forget why they entered but remember quickly. With dementia, a person loses track of the date and becomes lost even in familiar areas. It is also worth mentioning that a low mood, anxiety, or irritability is normal in the aging process.

With dementia, the person usually becomes withdrawn, easily irritable, sad, and frightened. I become concerned when a person forgets an entire story or part of a story. For example, a family member of mine was telling a story about a bike path he made and completely forgot my daughter was there to see it. Even when reminded, he could not recall that event. When I am asked about normal aging versus dementia, I often state that if your keys are lost, and you can backtrack and find them, there is no concern. If you lose your keys because you put them in the refrigerator, there may be a problem.

There is also a condition known as mild cognitive impairment (MCI), which is a minor but recognizable decline in cognitive abilities, such as memory and thinking skills. A person with MCI is at a higher risk of developing Alzheimer's disease or related dementia. Of people sixty-five years and older, approximately 15–20 percent have MCI. MCI is not "a little bit" of dementia. I hear that term used often and can tell you there is no such thing as a little bit of dementia. It is like saying someone is a little bit pregnant. You either are or are not pregnant, just like you either have dementia or you do not.

Although I have extensive experience with dementia, I do not claim to have all the answers. As with anything in life, there is always more to learn. Some of the methods I have used may not be suitable for your situation or may seem incorrect to you. I am aware of my imperfections and can admit I have made mistakes in handling some situations. If an approach I describe feels improper, just know, my decisions have been guided by a desire to help and are based on what I felt was right in that moment. We all make mistakes along this journey, despite our very best efforts, so remember to be patient with yourself. I hope you find these stories interesting and informative, as well as learn some strategies that are useful for your situation.

# ACKNOWLEDGEMENTS

I would like to thank my husband, Ryan Johnson, for encouraging and supporting me while I wrote this book. There were many late nights of discussing difficult client cases and contemplation of the flow of the book. He also read each chapter after I finished and reminded me of some facts I had forgotten. I would also like to thank my daughter, Alana Elizabeth Camille Campos, for keeping me on my toes. Also, thank you to everyone who believed in me throughout the years. You know who you are. Finally, thank you for those who doubted me. You made me stronger.

# ABBREVIATIONS

| | |
|---|---|
| AAA: | American Automobile Association |
| ABN: | Advance Beneficiary Notice |
| ACA: | Affordable Care Act |
| ADL: | activities of daily living |
| ADR: | Alternative Dispute Resolution |
| ADRD: | Alzheimer's disease related neurocognitive disorders |
| AL: | assisted living |
| AOTA: | American Occupation Therapy Association |
| APS: | Adult Protective Services |
| CCRC: | continuing care retirement community |
| CHAMPVA: | Civilian Health and Medical Program of the Department of Veterans Affairs |
| CMI: | chronic mental illness |
| COPD: | chronic obstructive pulmonary disease |
| CPR: | cardiopulmonary resuscitation |
| CT: | computerized tomography |
| CVA: | cerebral vascular accident |
| DNR: | do not resuscitate |
| EEG: | electroencephalogram |
| FAST: | Functional Assessment Staging |
| FHA: | Federal Housing Administration |
| FPOA: | financial power of attorney |

| | |
|---|---|
| FSA: | flexible spending account |
| FTD: | frontotemporal dementia |
| GDS: | Global Deterioration Scale for Assessment of Primary Degenerative Dementia |
| GEP: | General Enrollment Period |
| GFI: | ground fault interrupter |
| HECM: | Home Equity Conversion Mortgage |
| HMO: | health maintenance organization |
| HUD: | Department of Housing and Urban Development |
| IADL: | instrumental activities of daily living |
| ICU: | intensive care unit |
| IEP: | Initial Enrollment Period |
| IL: | independent living |
| INR: | international normalized ratio |
| IV: | intravenous |
| LBD: | Lewy body dementia |
| MCI: | mild cognitive impairment |
| MRI: | magnetic resonance imaging |
| MSA: | Medical Savings Account |
| NOMNC: | Notice of Medicare Noncoverage |
| NPH: | normal pressure hydrocephalus |
| PACE: | Program of All-Inclusive Care for the Elderly |
| PCP: | primary care physician |
| PET: | positron emission tomography |
| PFFS: | Private Fee-For-Service |
| POA: | power of attorney |
| PPO: | Preferred Provider Organization |
| PSO: | Point-of-Service |
| PTSD: | posttraumatic stress disorder |
| REM: | rapid eye movement |
| SEP: | Special Enrollment Period |

| | |
|---|---|
| SNAP: | Supplemental Nutrition Assistance Program |
| SNF: | skilled nursing facility |
| SNP: | Special Needs Plan |
| SSI: | Supplemental Security Income |
| SSRIs: | selective serotonin reuptake inhibitors |
| TIA: | transient ischemic attack |
| TFL: | TRICARE for Life |
| UA: | urinalysis |
| UTI: | urinary tract infection |
| VA: | Veteran Affairs |

# CHAPTER 1:
# WHAT IS DEMENTIA?

If you have met one person with dementia, then you
have met one person with dementia.

—Anonymous

*Dementia* is a general term representing loss of memory,
language, problem-solving, and other cognitive abilities
that interfere with daily life and function. Dementia is not a
single disease. Think of dementia as an umbrella diagnosis,
under which there are specific diseases. Another umbrella
diagnosis is cancer. If a doctor diagnosed your loved one
with cancer, you would want to know what type, location,
and advancement of the disease. If a doctor diagnosed your
loved one with dementia, you should ask the type, know
how advanced it is, and the characteristics of that type of
dementia.

Dementia is not an uncommon disease, yet many people
do not understand the disease or are frightened by it.
Approximately 5.8 million Americans have been diagnosed

with Alzheimer's disease related neurocognitive disorders (ADRD). Based on the evolutionary rise of ADRD, prevalence is expected to grow to 13.8 million Americans by 2050. Despite the advancements in dementia research, there remains many unanswered questions. With exponential growth, dementia will affect someone you know at some point in your life. As if these numbers are not astonishing enough, the cost of dementia (health care and paid/unpaid caregiver support) for ADRD is approximately a quarter of a billion dollars. The cost is expected to expand to greater than $1.1 trillion by 2050. Time is another factor to consider. According to the Alzheimer's Association (2018), 18.5 billion hours of care was provided by informal caregivers. This means lost hours of work and time away from family to care for a loved one.

Studies suggest the optimal time to diagnose and intervene in terms of delaying decline is when cognitive disorders are still in mild stages. Early diagnosis and intervention may decrease the severity of behavioral and psychological symptoms associated with dementia. It also allows persons with dementia and their caregivers more time to establish support systems, seek education, understand treatment options, and plan. Unfortunately, dementia is often diagnosed beyond the mild, early stages. Approximately 30 percent of persons with dementia are diagnosed by their primary care provider. Coupled with a poor understanding of prognosis, disease progression is complicated by unnecessary emergency room visits, hospitalization, and aggressive medical interventions, which negatively impacts quality of life.

## HOW THE BRAIN WORKS

The brain is a very complex organ, with intricate wiring and serves many important functions. There are numerous books and articles about the brain, and as fascinating as it is, I am sticking to the basics for the purposes of this book.

The components of the brain are the *brainstem, cerebellum,* and *cerebrum.* The brainstem is the lower extension of the brain. Many functions for survival are in the brainstem, such as breathing, blood pressure, heart rhythms, and swallowing. The brainstem is also involved with communication within the brain and with other parts of the body. Ocular motion, hearing, balance, sleep cycles, facial sensations, and taste are just a few of the other functions served by the brainstem. The cerebellum is in the back of the brain. The cerebellum is responsible for fine motor movements in addition to rapid and repetitive movements, sense of equilibrium or balance, and control of the tone of muscles. The cerebrum forms the major portion of the brain and is divided into right and left hemispheres. Each hemisphere has a frontal, temporal, parietal, and occipital lobe. Within the temporal lobe is the limbic system, which is significantly impacted during the progression of Alzheimer's disease. Specific functions are controlled by each lobe. These lobes do not function alone but rather through a complex network with one another:

**Frontal Lobe.** Personality, behavior, emotions, judgment, problem solving, executive function, speech, and body movement

**Temporal Lobe.** Memory formation, hearing, sequencing, organization, language comprehension, emotion association

> **Limbic System.** Located immediately beneath the medial temporal lobe, and includes the hypothalamus (hormone management, body temperature regulation, appetite control, regulation of emotions, management of sexual behavior), part of the thalamus (regulation of consciousness, sleep, and alertness and communication of sensory signals), amygdala (memory processing, decision-making, emotional responses), and hippocampus (formation of new memories, associated with learning and emotions)

**Parietal Lobe.** Sensory processing (touch, pressure, pain, and temperature), hearing and visual perception, memory, navigation, and spatial and visual perception

**Occipital Lobe.** Functional vision, visual orientation, visual perception of color, light, and movement

## DEMENTIA

Depending on who you ask, there may be anywhere from 40–80 types of dementia, some of which are extremely rare. According to the Alzheimer's Association, the most prevalent types of Dementia are Lewy body dementia, Alzheimer's disease, frontotemporal dementia, and vascular dementia. Other less prevalent but normally occurring dementias include Huntington's disease, normal pressure hydrocephalus, posterior cortical atrophy, Parkinson's disease dementia, Creutzfeldt-Jakob disease, and Korsakoff dementia. A person can also have mixed dementia, meaning there is more than one type of dementia occurring simultaneously.

Since Alzheimer's disease is the most common form of dementia, I am going to describe brain changes that occur as the disease progresses. The descriptions of common signs and symptoms corresponding to the area of damage is useful material, as damage to these areas cause the same signs and symptoms regardless of the type of dementia.

## ALZHEIMER'S DISEASE

Alzheimer's disease accounts for 60–70 percent of all dementias. The brain changes with Alzheimer's disease are well known; however, the cause of these changes is still researched heavily. Abnormal clusters of proteins (plaque) build up between the nerve cells and twisted tangles of proteins inside of the nerve cell cause destruction of the nerves and cell death. The plaques and tangles impair the transmission of electrical messages between the neurons. As nerve cells die, the brain shrinks, and brain function is impaired. If you were to look at a scan of a normal brain next to the brain of a person with advanced Alzheimer's, you would observe a much smaller brain in the person with Alzheimer's disease. Changes in the brain generally occur in a predictable manner as each area of the brain is affected. After the limbic system is affected, the disease progresses to the parietal lobe, followed by the temporal lobe, then the occipital lobe, and finally the hypothalamus, frontal lobe, and cortexes.

Often, the first symptom of Alzheimer's disease is an alteration in short-term memory. This occurs because of the changes occurring in the limbic system, specifically the hippocampus. As mentioned, the hippocampus is responsible for processing memory. This would include transitioning short-term memories into long-term memories. When this part of the brain is damaged, short-term memories are not able to be stored as long-term memories. Therefore, we see forgetfulness as one of the first symptoms of Alzheimer's disease. With that, the ability to learn new information is extremely difficult, as is the ability to follow directions. This area of the brain is responsible for spatial processing, which provides the ability to know where objects are in space and on the body. As such, this area controls the ability to navigate one's environment. This area of the brain is also important for time awareness, sensory inputs from the skin, and language. When this area of the brain is affected, impairments with hand-eye coordination, writing, mathematics, and perception of objects, as well as language disorders, are likely to be seen. This can include difficulty interpreting and learning words and difficulty recognizing objects by tactile stimuli. Drawing abilities and self-care activities, such as dressing, are likely to be impacted. Reaching for an item may become difficult due to inability to correctly estimate the object's distance from oneself. There can also be a lack of awareness of sensation, such as difficulty discerning hot water from cold water.

The temporal lobe is involved in processing sensory input, retention of visual memory, language comprehension, and emotional association. The temporal lobe communicates with the hippocampus to process visual memory and formulate long-term memories. The temporal lobe is also involved in auditory perception, which allows sensory information to be translated into meaningful communication. The temporal lobe is thought to be involved in encoding declarative long-term memory, which is the process by which memories are consciously stored in the brain. When this area of the brain is affected, there is a disruption of auditory sensation and perception, which can cause hearing loss. The ability to recognize faces may be affected. Visual-perception distortion, impaired organization of verbal stimuli, difficulty with language comprehension, impaired memory, and altered personality are all possible complications from damage to the temporal lobe.

The occipital lobe is largely responsible for visual acuity, which is a highly complex process. The occipital lobe maps the visual environment, which helps with spatial and visual memory. This allows you to scan a visual field and connected frames of information to form a visual memory. This lobe also transmits visual information to other parts of the brain to help encode memories and assimilate to respond to information from the surrounding world. The occipital lobe is associated with visuospatial processing, distance, and depth perception, object and face recognition, and color determination. Damage to his area of the brain can cause visual deficits, such as mild blindness and difficulty identifying colors. Your loved one may have more difficulty recognizing your face or remember you as someone else from their past. There is an increased difficulty in recognizing words and objects. I have seen clients who pick up a television remote and think it is a telephone, which also occurs with damage to the occipital lobe.

The hypothalamus is located in the limbic layer and is near the hippocampus. Although the hypothalamus is small, it plays an imperative role in many important functions, such as hormone regulation, appetite control, management of sexual behavior, sleep, controlling emotional responses, and regulating body temperature. The main symptoms correlated to a damaged hypothalamus in Alzheimer's disease is body-temperature changes, weight fluctuations, behavioral changes, and alterations in sleep cycle. Generally, when a person has entered middle- to late-stage Alzheimer's, it is common to feel cold and have difficulty getting warm. (This will be important to remember when we discuss difficulty with bathing later in this book.) I have witnessed weight fluctuations occur in two different ways. First when the appetite regulator causes a person to feel hungry most of the time. I had a gentleman I cared for wake up around 7:00 a.m. and ask for breakfast. I would make him a complete breakfast. He would say he was tired and wanted to lie down. An hour later he was awake and was ready for breakfast. He usually ate three breakfasts a day. He would also eat several lunches and dinners. He had no awareness; he just ate and would tell me how hungry he was. I also had a gentleman I cared for who would eat until he vomited. His brain had minimal ability to regulate his hunger. Unfortunately, his son did not see he needed more help, and I would find him lying in bed with vomit all over him. This is not a common occurrence but can happen.

Many family members are concerned about overeating, especially if there are weight issues. I often encourage eating in this phase if there are not immediate health concerns, because as the disease progresses, the opposite happens with appetite regulation. A person with advanced Alzheimer's does not have an awareness of hunger and will refuse meals. Weight loss is expected. I have seen family members force food during this phase, which can cause more harm than good. This change is normal as Alzheimer's continues to strip away brain function. Behavioral changes are generally sexual in nature when the hypothalamus is affected. The ability to distinguish between appropriate and inappropriate behaviors is impaired. This can be very concerning to family members and caregivers, but there are methods to diffuse behaviors, which will be discussed in later chapters. Lastly, it is not uncommon for a person with Alzheimer's disease to stay awake for days at a time and then sleep for twenty-four to forty-eight hours. There can also be difficulty discerning between days and nights, and the sleep-wake cycle can be reversed. Tactics to keep your own sanity will be discussed in later chapters.

Concurrently with changes to the hypothalamus are changes to the frontal lobe and to the motor and somatosensory cortex, which are located between the frontal lobe and the parietal lobe. The simultaneous changes that are occurring in these areas explains the dramatic changes seen in the middle and late stages of Alzheimer's disease. The frontal lobe controls important cognitive skills, such as problem solving, judgment, executive function, and social behavior. Part of the frontal lobe is also responsible for primary motor function, which allows for the ability to consciously move muscles. Some people with Alzheimer's will have involuntary movements, such as myoclonus, as a result. Another area of the frontal lobe, Broca's area, is linked to language comprehension, speech-associated motions, language fluidity, and speech production. Damage to the frontal lobe can result in a decrease in attention and ability to focus, personality or mood changes, slower information processing, difficulty with social interaction, and inability to plan or execute plans, as well as cause multiple impediments with language and speech.

As the name implies, the motor cortex is responsible for motor movements. These purposeful movements include everything from large to small muscles and even swallowing motions. This area controls impulses that pass down the spinal cord and control the execution of movement, motor control in preparing for movements, and the planning and coordination of movement. Damage to this area is seen on the side opposite of the area affected, meaning damage to the right hemisphere is seen on the left side of the body and vice versa. Damage can include involuntary muscle contractions, spastic muscles, and loss of fine motor skills. Movements are less coordinated, and the thought process for muscle movement is delayed.

The somatosensory cortex is responsible for processing somatic sensations, meaning sensations from the body instead of sensations from specialized sense organs such as the eyes or ears. The somatosensory receptors detect touch, proprioception (the position of the body in space), nociception (such as pain), and temperature. Damage to this area causes decreased sensory thresholds, causing an inability to distinguish aspects of tactile stimuli or the ability to identify objects by touch. Impairment to this area also affects the quality of pain sensations and the ability to identify the location of a painful stimulus, as well as the ability to know the difference between hot and cold temperatures.

## VASCULAR DEMENTIA

Vascular dementia is believed to be the second most common dementia, accounting for 15–20 percent of all dementias. Vascular dementia is the result of reduced blood flow to the brain, leading to deprivation of oxygen and nutrients. Often, vascular dementia occurs as the result of a stroke (cerebral vascular accident [CVA]) or transient ischemic attack (TIA). A stroke or TIA does not guarantee vascular dementia but does increase the risk. Other factors that increase the risk of vascular dementia include diabetes, high blood pressure, high cholesterol, and smoking; these factors increase the risk of decreased vascularization.

The severity of the disease depends on the extent of damage to blood vessels and subsequent circulation. The symptoms also depend on the area of the brain where damage occurred. Earlier I discussed the function of different parts of the brain. Corresponding effects would be directly related to the area of the brain that is damaged. For example, if the frontal lobe is affected, we would expect vascular dementia to present with personality changes, loss of control of emotions, abnormal behaviors, difficulty with language, and difficulty with problem solving and judgment.

Common consequences of vascular cognitive impairment include *agnosia*, *aphasia*, and *apraxia*. Agnosia is the inability to recognize familiar objects, even if there are no sensory deficits. Aphasia is loss of the ability to communicate. With expressive aphasia, a person understands the words that are said but cannot express themselves appropriately. With receptive aphasia, a person is having difficulty receiving the message being communicated. Apraxia is difficulty with physical movement even with normal physical functioning.

## FRONTOTEMPORAL DEMENTIA

Frontotemporal dementia (FTD) affects, as the name suggests, the frontal and temporal lobes. FTD is believed to account for about 10–20 percent of all dementias. The frontal and temporal lobes atrophy (shrink) as the disease progresses. FTD is often misdiagnosed as Alzheimer's disease or a psychiatric disorder; however, FTD usually occurs at a younger age.

The most common symptoms associated with FTD are behavioral changes and problems with speech and language. Inappropriate sexual behavior, lack of empathy, apathy, lack of judgment, lack of inhibition, repetitive compulsive behavior, and a decline in personal hygiene are also common with FTD. Other signs include difficulty in using and understanding written and spoken language, sentence construction errors, and difficulty naming items.

The first time I cared for a person with FTD was when I was working in a hospice inpatient unit. A gentleman was transferred to the hospice unit because his family was having challenges managing his behavior at home. The purpose of his admission was medication management, with the hopes of controlling his behaviors and his returning home. My patient was a Baptist minister, and his family was devoted to the church. His FTD presented with the use of profane language and inappropriate sexual inuendo. His family was devastated and embarrassed. I cared for another woman who was a business owner and conservative. Her FTD presented in her fifties when she displayed inappropriate sexual behavior in public. She would expose herself to strangers and was posting comments on social media indicating she was wealthy, has dementia, and is looking for a mate. I am sure you can see why FTD is misdiagnosed for a psychiatric disorder.

## LEWY BODY DEMENTIA

Lewy body dementia (LBD) is also a commonly misdiagnosed disease. It is estimated that 3–7 percent of dementia cases are due to Lewy bodies, although true prevalence is probably higher. LBD is the result of cells containing an aggregation of a protein that overwhelms the cell's normal functions and leads to cell death with subsequent loss of nerve cells. Lewy bodies are the accumulation of proteins seen in the cell. Lewy bodies are also present with Parkinson's disease. The motor symptoms associated with LBD are uniform with Parkinson's.

The presentation of LBD includes cognitive, motor, and psychiatric symptoms, as well as autonomic dysfunction.

Memory may be intact but other aspects of cognition are affected. Common cognitive impairments include deficits with executive function, difficulty recognizing familiar people or objects, reduced attention, slow thinking, and alterations in cognition. LBD can be challenging to diagnose because there can be very lucid days, where cognitive function is normal, alternating with obvious signs of cognitive impairment. If memory is also intact, it is difficult to diagnose cognitive impairment.

I saw the variations of cognition when I worked in hospice. We had one patient who was declining, but the progression of the illness was difficult to put on paper. When she had a good day, she did not appear to be appropriate for hospice services. Her good days would alternate with days where she was completely bedbound, lacked verbal communication, and experienced extreme fatigue.

Motor symptoms with LBD may be subtle at first and may begin later in the disease process. Motor symptoms include reduced facial expression (frozen face), soft voice, stiffness, difficulty with balance, falls, slowed movements, and tremors at rest. If these symptoms are present and there is no indication of dementia, the person may have Parkinson's as opposed to LBD.

Psychiatric symptoms are a classic presentation with LBD. Visual hallucinations (seeing something that is not real) occur in up to 80 percent of people with LBD. Apathy, anxiety, depression, and aggressive behaviors can occur. Rapid eye movement (REM) sleeping behavior disorder presents with acting out dreams. The person may scream, thrash, punch, and kick while sleeping. A normal sleep pattern consists of sleep paralysis during REM sleep to keep us from acting out our dreams. This disorder can lead to harm for the person or their bed partner.

Severe autonomic dysfunction may also occur in LBD. Symptoms associated with autonomic dysfunction include orthostatic hypotension (lowered blood pressure when sitting or standing), urinary incontinence, constipation, and erectile dysfunction. It can also present with impaired sense of smell, excessive sweating alternating with scaly skin, and drooling. The biggest concern with autonomic dysfunction is the increased risk of falls. A person with LBD may become dizzy when going from a lying position to sitting and from a sitting position to a standing position. It is important these movements are carried out slowly.

Medication management with LBD proves to be most challenging. With the multitude of distressing symptoms, medications may be desired to improve quality of life. Unfortunately, a person with LBD is highly sensitive to medications, such as antipsychotics and antidepressants. Common classes of medication to treat behaviors cause a paradoxical effect, making behaviors and hallucinations worse. This is the reason I push for an exact diagnosis. Knowing what kind of dementia is present is important later in the disease from a medication-management standpoint.

## OBTAINING A DEMENTIA DIAGNOSIS

The Global Deterioration Scale for Assessment of Primary Degenerative Dementia (GDS), developed by Dr. Barry Reisberg, provides an outline for the stages of cognitive function for those with a primary degenerative dementia. There are seven stages, with stage 1 being no cognitive decline and stage 7 being severe dementia. In my experience, it is not uncommon for a person to be diagnosed with dementia until they are in stage four, which is moderate cognitive decline or mild dementia. I have also met clients in stage five, which is moderately severe cognitive decline, when diagnosed with dementia. I have met many physicians who fail to properly assess for dementia, which leads to late diagnosis. A person with mild dementia may present well and answer questions as though cognitive impairment is not present; however, the answers to those questions are likely inaccurate. For this reason, people with mild dementia are known as the Great Foolers, as they have compensated for lost short-term memories. I have found pushing physicians to complete cognitive testing, rather than ask questions where an answer cannot be verified, can be particularly challenging. It is worth pushing for a diagnosis, as the best time to initiate medication specific to dementia is earlier in the disease process. Later in this book I will discuss obtaining the correct dementia diagnosis.

Even though these are the basics with dementia, I realize it is a lot to take in. You may need to reference back to this chapter as you go through the book. In fact, you may find it helpful to reread the material as you gain more information to help assimilate your newfound knowledge.

# Chapter 2:
# I Think My Mom Has
# Dementia

It is not how much you do, but how much
love you put in the doing.

—Mother Teresa

Sitting in a coffee shop during a warm October day, I met with Shirley's son to discuss his situation and determine if I would be of any assistance. The inquiry started with an email titled "I think my mom has dementia." Dave explained some behaviors that he could not make sense of and was not sure what they meant. He indicated that prior to his father's death a year ago he did notice some impairment with short-term memories, but he brushed it off as part of the aging process. Dave, a man in his sixties, put his work life on hold after his father's death to care for his mother, despite health care being far from his area of expertise. Now in her late eighties, Shirley was living alone in the home her and her husband had resided in for the past twenty years. Neighbors were reporting seeing Shirley in street in the middle of the night, and there were frequent calls from the local police to indicate she called in a forced entry into her home. Dave stated some of the officers were familiar with Shirley and her frequent calls. I knew something was wrong, but also I knew a thorough evaluation was needed to start putting pieces together. A week later I had the pleasure to meet Shirley in her private home.

Shirley looked much like a diva, with her perfectly color-coordinated outfit and sparkly hat. She had red lipstick and rose blush, which she wore whether she had plans or not. She spoke with a Southern twang and exuded poise and confidence. She seemed to enjoy my assessment as it put her in the spotlight. Her physical assessment was normal. She appeared very healthy. She had been prescribed two medications: one medication was for memory and the other was for hypothyroidism. She was reportedly non-compliant with both, which I confirmed when she could not bring the bottles to me because she did not know where they were. The Mini-Mental State Examination indicated mild cognitive impairment (MCI). The Mini-Cog, which is a short screening for cognitive impairment, indicated dementia. It was evident there were deficits with short-term memory, concentration, and reasoning.

My initial assessment also includes determining if behaviors are present. Since Dave indicated the police were being called often, I asked Shirley if anything in her life was bothering her. Shirley indicated a woman had been entering her house without an invitation. She stated the woman is a locksmith and has been making keys and handing the keys out to random people. Shirley felt the woman and her daughter were entering her home as they wished. The two women reportedly stole items, such as glasses and books. Shirley felt the women were taking these items to get under her skin. She also revealed she has twenty-seven clothes hangers that do not have clothing because the women stole clothing. She thought the women borrowed her clothes, brought them back, and put her clothing back on the hangers. Shirley always kept her purse close and even slept with it. She refused to sleep in her room due to fear of intruders, so she slept on a couch in the front room of the house. When she would call the police, she was told they could not do anything unless the women were in her home. Although the information is not factual, it was very real to her. She lived in constant fear. Trying to reason with her would be fruitless, so it was important to listen and validate her feelings while making her feel safe.

Dave indicated his mother had not been to the doctor in quite some time. He also indicated legal documents, such as power of attorney (POA), were not in place. Dave requested care management services to ensure adequate healthcare coverage and in-home care one day per week to allow Shirley to get out and run errands, as well as have companionship. Shirley started receiving in-home care but refused to leave her home due to concerns of strangers entering her home while away. She rarely even went outside to check the mail. It was apparent her paranoia and delusions were affecting her everyday life.

Shirley visited her primary care physician (PCP), Dr. Sharma, shortly after my initial evaluation for an overall assessment and to have blood tests conducted. The results from labs indicated her thyroid was extremely underactive, which confirmed that she had not been taking her thyroid medication. Dr. Sharma advised her to restart her thyroid medication. He checked other labs that coincide with conditions that can affect cognition, such as vitamin B-12 levels. The medication Aricept (donepezil) was started as dementia was suspected. An MRI of the brain was ordered, and Dr. Sharma recommended routine health-care maintenance, such as a hearing exam and a vision screening.

Her son and I worked as a team. He ensured the recommended tests and exams were scheduled, while I was responsible for her medication and physician communication. Since she was home alone most of the time, I used a locked, electronic medication box. An alarm would go off and provide the medication Shirley was to take. She took her medication about half of the time, which was progress. Over the course of the next month, her compliance with medication continued to improve.

Dave and I went to the follow-up appointment with Dr. Sharma to review the results of the MRI and follow-up labs. Shirley's thyroid level remained low, so the dose of her medication was adjusted. Her labs also showed renal impairment, which was likely the result of dehydration. Dr. Sharma indicated the MRI was mildly abnormal. He stated Shirley's cognition may improve when thyroid levels are stabilized and with an increase in Aricept. Dr. Sharma stated he wanted to see Shirley in two to three months.

While addressing Shirley's medical care, there was also a focus on getting her legal affairs in order. Dave was able to retain the services of an attorney that came to the home to have documents signed. Shirley signed the documents and the family finally had ability to step in and help as her life was changing.

**LEGAL CONSIDERATIONS**

Often, legal documents have not been started when I become involved. A part of my role is to be proactive and assist in getting legal affairs in order. Having a dementia diagnosis means there are immediate and necessary steps that need to be implemented for estate and long-term-care planning if they have not been completed previously. If documents are in place, it is also important to review documents to ensure all considerations have been addressed. It is commonly believed that a dementia diagnosis terminates your ability to execute a will or trust or establish long-term-care planning. The diagnosis does not automatically indicate a person has lost the ability to have legal capacity to sign documents. However, once a person has been determined to lack capacity to make appropriate decisions, the ability to execute documents is no longer available.

I always recommend getting legal affairs in order as soon as possible. Once a person has significant cognitive impairment and is no longer able to execute documents, legal decision-making becomes complicated. In the United States, a hierarchy for a health-care surrogate, also known as proxy, indicates the order of priority of family and friends who can serve as a decision maker in the absence of a POA or court appointment. If a proxy cannot be identified or there are concerns about the surrogate's ability to make sound decisions, legal proceedings may be required to provide protection to the vulnerable adult. This process is expensive and labor intensive. It is best to save the time and money and be prepared prior to any complications.

Medical directives are important for everyone to have, regardless of age or medical conditions, but are extremely important for a person diagnosed with dementia. Medical directives include health-care power of attorney, mental health power of attorney (varies by state), living will, and a do not resuscitate (DNR)/prehospital medical care directive order if applicable.

A health-care POA is an agent that is appointed to make medical decisions when a person is no longer able to direct their own care. Depending on what state you live in, POA documents may not be inclusive of mental-health powers, and a mental health

POA is needed. It is imperative to know if the extra POA is needed, especially if the person with dementia develops behaviors and needs inpatient treatment. A living will provides direction on type of care that is desired if a person can no longer speak for herself. Living-will directives include decisions on comfort care, cardiopulmonary resuscitation (CPR), and artificially administered food and fluids. Medical directive documents can be completed through an elder law attorney or can be downloaded from your state's attorney general website and completed without an attorney but would require a notary. A DNR is a directive indicating a person does not want life-sustaining treatment, such as CPR and defibrillation. A DNR does not mean "do not treat," which is a common misconception. If a person with a DNR has a fall, for example, and needs treatment, going to the hospital to receive care is completely appropriate. Check your state's specific requirements for life care planning.

Directives related to finances are also important to put into place. Depending on the complexity of assets, the expense of an attorney may be well worth the cost. The National Academy of Elder Law Attorneys is a great resource to find an attorney in your area that can be of assistance. A financial power of attorney (FPOA) is a legal document that allows an agent the authority to make financial decisions on behalf of a person who is not able to do so themselves. An FPOA is also referred to as a general POA. Check your state's guidelines for specific information on the use of an FPOA. If you carry out an FPOA without the assistance of an attorney, you will likely need to ensure it is notarized.

Deciding on who should be responsible to fill the role of a POA is an important one. While most people choose a family member or close friend to carry out this role, others turn to a third party. Most commonly a licensed fiduciary is hired to serve in the role of health-care POA and/or FPOA. A fiduciary can be hired by an individual without the need for court proceedings.

Over the course of the next couple of months, there were many changes, and the care team grew. Shirley's eye exam resulted in the discovery of cataracts to both eyes. Cataract surgery was recommended; however, Shirley's eyes were too dry to schedule the surgery. She was given two different eye drops that she needed to administer frequently throughout the day. After the eye appointment, I met with Dave and Shirley to discuss the plan. I recall Shirley looking at the bottles of eye drops, asking what they were for and Dave explaining the purpose and frequency of administering the eye drops. Shirley stated she understood and less than two minutes later asked, "What are these for?" Dave went through the entire explanation again. This cycle occurred several times until I told Dave his mother is not capable of learning new information and cannot be responsible for ensuring the drops are being given appropriately. Dave mentioned he would call each time the drops were needed, but that still would not assure she administered the drops. I talked to Dave about getting some additional care in place to confirm she is getting the drops, while monitoring her overall cognition. After evaluating the need, Dave decided to initiate eleven hours of care every day until her follow-up appointment. The additional hours allowed the team a wide viewpoint of the extent of Shirley's dementia.

After initiating additional care, Shirley returned to see Dr. Sharma as requested. While the doctor was in the room, Shirley turned to me and stated she does not understand why she must see her doctor because he does not do anything for her. She stated she does not even like him. I pointed to the doctor to let her know he was in the room. Her demeanor completely changed. Dr. Sharma asked Shirley to walk to the table for an examination. As she grabbed his hands, she started to dance with him. She was very happy and seemed to forget the comments she just made. After giving general updates, the real conversations started. I asked Shirley to tell her doctor about the women who are trying to come into her home. She told him an elaborate story, which seemingly was not factual, however, completely real to her. Dr. Sharma was also made aware of new behaviors that have been noted since her having increased care. Shirley was getting lost in her home. She would frequently ask her caregivers where different rooms in the home were. She was found urinating in the closet, likely because she did not know where the bathroom was. She also did not have a full awareness of when she needed to urinate, and it was reported she was occasionally incontinent of bladder. I also made him aware of her recent decreased appetite and weight loss. I asked Dr. Sharma to add a urinalysis (UA) to her labs to rule out a urinary tract infection (UTI).

The lab technician took Shirley into the bathroom and provided step-by-step instructions on what was needed. While she was in the bathroom, Dave spoke to Dr. Sharma to inquire if Shirley has dementia and if so, how far has it progressed. Dr. Sharma stated she has "early, severe dementia." I believe Dave only heard the early part and did not seem to have an awareness of how severe her dementia was. It did not help that Dr. Sharma did not want to elaborate on her disease process and seemed ambivalent about the subject in general. He did switch her to another medication, Namzaric, which is a combination therapy drug consisting of memantine and donepezil (common medications used to treat dementia). Dr. Sharma was optimistic the new medication would help Shirley's cognition.

Shirley had been in the bathroom for longer than expected for a UA. I went into the bathroom to check on her. She was standing in the corner of the bathroom without any clothing from the waist down, including shoes. She had a puddle of urine underneath her. She was able to get enough of a sample in the cup to run a UA. She indicated she urinated on her panties and could not wear them. After I cleaned the floor and helped her get dressed, I put her panties into an empty urine sample cup and gave it to her caregiver to wash once they returned home. Shirley came out of the bathroom without anybody knowing what happened, and she maintained her dignity.

As suspected, Shirley did have a urinary tract infection. She was started on antibiotics, and her symptoms of decreased appetite and urinary incontinence improved. Shirley started to slowly gain weight back. The successes were short-lived.

During the hours Shirley was home alone, she sustained a fall on tile and was found on the floor with blood surrounding her. She was taken to the hospital, where it was discovered she had a subdural hematoma, which is the presence of blood between the brain and the membrane around the brain. Since she was stable, the plan was to watch and follow up with a neurologist. A post-hospitalization appointment was made with Dr. Sharma. He ordered a repeat CT scan to compare to the CT in the hospital to ensure the bleed is stable. If it were not, she would have to see a neurosurgeon. Thankfully, the CT showed the bleed was stable and it eventually resolved without intervention. I always took the opportunity in these visits to have the doctor reiterate what is necessary. We talked about Shirley's delusions and cognitive impairment. Dr. Sharma stated the level of impairment and falls; twenty-four-hour care is needed immediately. Lastly, I asked Dr. Sharma to include the diagnosis of dementia on his visit note so a claim to the long-term-care insurance company can be started. Dave agreed to twenty-four-hour care, but knew it was not financially sustainable, so the goal was to move Shirley into a memory-care facility.

Shirley received twenty-four-hour care, which consisted of twelve-hour shifts, with each caregiver reporting to the next. I continued to monitor medications and oversee the care. With the additional care, new insights were obtained, which added even more complexity to Shirley's care. I received a call one morning from the nighttime caregiver, who reported that Shirley became very angry and attacked her. She grabbed and pulled her by the hair and scratched her a couple of times. The caregiver was shaken up after the incident. I received another report that Shirley asked the caregiver to look for something in the closet and when she did, Shirley pushed her into the closet and shut the door. She was staying awake for days at a time and would then sleep an entire day.

During this time, Dave was looking for a memory-care facility for his mom. He identified one he thought would be a good fit for Shirley. I updated Dave on behaviors that were emerging. I made him aware his mom cannot go to a facility with these behaviors as the facility would likely send her to an acute psychiatric facility to stabilize her and potentially ask her to not return if they feel she is threat to other residents. I suggested getting a psychiatrist to get medications started and allow time for adjustments before she moved. Dave agreed, and a mobile psychiatrist visited Shirley. The psychiatrist started her on Seroquel (quetiapine), which is a common antipsychotic medication used for dementia with behaviors. There were a couple of minor adjustments to the medication, but the right dose was determined, and she was stable enough to move into the memory-care facility. Shirley continued to have caregivers she was familiar with for a couple hours a day to help her adjust to her new setting. She seemed to adjust well, and caregiving services were stopped.

Shirley demonstrated some behaviors, not nearly as severe, with the care staff at the facility. The change in environment was overwhelming. During my initial visits, she talked about her husband and stated he left her for another woman. She said he found a younger woman and married her, but his new wife ended up leaving him. This story was consistently told for several months. She would also talk about Dave, indicating he has been causing harm to others and is in jail. None of these stories were accurate, but they were real in her mind. As time went on, those stories faded away. Shirley enjoyed talking about her family and interactions she had with her parents and siblings; however, she thought the interactions occurred recently. As her disease progressed, her only conversation topic was of family life on the farm. She enjoyed telling these stories and laughed often when telling them. She would tell the same story several times over the course of the conversation. I entered her world by asking questions and engaging in conversations as if her recollections were in the present time.

Shirley's condition continued to deteriorate. There were many decisions that needed to be made to proactively ensure proper care. The family agreed a DNR would be appropriate. There were many conversations about disease progression and eventually hospice services were initiated. Shirley gave everyone a scare shortly after going onto hospice services; it appeared she was at the very end. She ended up pulling through that. She was on hospice services for a year, but eventually hospice did graduate her. She was gaining weight, starting to walk again, and seemed to be thriving.

**HOSPICE**

I have met many people who believe hospice is a place or care that is intended for the last days of life. Hospice is in fact a philosophy for end-of-life care and can be provided anywhere a person considers home. A physician certifies the condition is terminal and if the disease follows its normal course, there is a life expectancy of six months or less. Unfortunately, many people start hospice services just days or weeks prior to death and do not fully benefit from the services. Since we do not have a crystal ball, we do not truly know when a person will die. It is a best guess. I have seen quite a few people on hospice longer than six months, not because they are abusing the system but because there is no way to know. If there is a continued decline and certain criteria are met, a person can remain on hospice longer than six months.

I strongly advocate for hospice services when a terminal diagnosis is received, aggressive treatment is not wanted, and quality of life is the most important factor. There continues to be many misconceptions about hospice. Hospice supports your loved one through the decline and can provide monitoring, intervention for complications, education, and many levels of support. Hospice patients are examined at regular frequencies and some patients on hospice are taken off service for an extended prognosis.

Shirley remained at the memory-care facility, and although the disease was progressing, she was stable. During my visits, she would be in a wheelchair as she was no longer able to walk. She spoke very few words. Shirley was not able to put sentences together, and when she tried, the words did not go together or did not make sense. Shirley was not able to feed herself, so staff took over that role. In my experience, this phase of dementia can last several years. There are several scales that assist in understanding where a person is with their dementia. One useful scale, mentioned earlier, is the Global Deterioration Scale for Assessment of Primary Degenerative Dementia (GDS). Based on the GDS, Shirley was stage 7, which indicates very severe cognitive decline or severe dementia. The Functional Assessment Staging (FAST) scale is widely used by hospice organizations to grade the deterioration of dementia. Stage 7 is further broken down to account for the subtle changes indicating cognitive decline. Shirley was at stage 7C; however, she continued to maintain a stable weight and was without complications of dementia, such as wounds and infections.

Unfortunately, the coronavirus, or COVID-19, led to changes in my role with Shirley. I was not granted entry into the memory-care facility for many months. Once the facility determined it was safe, I was able to visit with Shirley in her room. She seemed a little more fatigued but was stable. She was putting on weight and needing bigger clothes. At one point, she had a severe reaction to an antibiotic for a urinary tract infection and ended up in the hospital. I was granted permission to see her in the hospital and provide information to the staff on Shirley's history and characteristics of her dementia. Shirley spends her days watching television in her room and interacting with staff at the facility, where she is receiving total care. The end stage of her dementia is lasting longer than most people experience and may continue for several years. Only time will tell, but until then, she continues to enjoy talking about life on the farm and is content being back in her childhood.

# CHAPTER 3:
# A DEMENTIA DIAGNOSIS ALONE IS NOT ENOUGH

Remember . . . The person with dementia is not
GIVING you a hard time. The person with dementia
is HAVING a hard time.

—Anonymous

At first glance, Margaret, who was a petite ninety-two-year-old woman, was the quintessential sweet old lady. I was asked to assess her and arrange in-home care after a temporary guardian, appointed by the court, was put into place over concerns of Margaret's ability to care for herself safely. She was made aware of my visit prior to my arrival but was suspicious nonetheless. She viewed me from a bedroom window near the front door. She then walked to the front door and released a series of six locks. Her screen door had an additional two locks. After I entered, she went through the process of locking her doors.

Sensing her extreme paranoia, I kept conversation light and tried to get a feeling of how to best gain information. She had difficulty staying still. She walked from the living room to the kitchen to her room and back around again. She was calm while pacing the house. When she was not distracted with pacing, her communication was appropriate. Margaret was able to engage in discussion about current events, which gave the impression of her being oriented. Her demeanor changed and did not seem to be related to an occurrence or trigger.

Margaret displayed a wide array of emotions, as well as crying spells, severe sleep disturbance, agitation, verbal disruption, delusions, and hallucinations. There was no predictability to her behaviors, and shifting of emotions could occur rapidly. The first indication of an issue occurred during a normal conversation about politics. Margaret heard the air conditioning turn on, which prompted an immediate emotional response. She asked me to be very quiet and appeared frightened. She told me there was a man that had been entering her home at random times but now seems to have moved into the attic. She stated the man was dropping "ding-a-lings" from the air conditioning vents. She described the "ding-a-lings" as small, furry creatures with long nails that could be heard scratching on the floor. The creatures are not human or animal, according to Margaret. She stated the creatures made a loud screeching noise when released from the attic. These creatures also would attack her dog, biting his ankles. Margaret had a diagnosis of dementia with behavioral disturbance. The type of dementia was not identified, which would have been helpful.

## OBTAINING THE CORRECT DEMENTIA DIAGNOSIS

Dementia can be reversible or irreversible. Determining reversible causes for alterations in cognition is the first step in a obtaining a dementia diagnosis. With reversible dementia, the cause can be treated, and improvement is seen. One of the most common causes of reversible dementia is hypothyroidism. Vitamin and mineral deficiencies, depression, medication side effects, infections, and metabolic disorders can also be a culprit. If cognitive issues continue, despite ruling out or correcting issues, further investigation is needed. Dementia may also be present in addition to the conditions mentioned. For example, a person diagnosed with dementia, who is also noted to have thyroid disease, is treated for hypothyroidism, and cognition improves, despite the irreversible disease of dementia. Cognitive improvement would, however, be transient.

There are several tests that assist in diagnosing dementia, such as magnetic resonance imaging (MRI), positron emission tomography (PET) scan, computerized tomography (CT) scan, electroencephalogram (EEG), and neuropsychological examinations. Some, or all, of these tests may be ordered to understand the cause of cognitive impairment.

These results can be analyzed, and a diagnosis can be provided. It is important to understand that a diagnosis is based on evaluation of symptoms and testing but is not definitive. The only definitive way to diagnosis the type of dementia is on autopsy.

You may ask, "Why is it important to get a specific dementia diagnosis?" The right diagnosis is imperative in the management of symptoms and improving quality of life for several reasons. The first reason is it allows loved ones to prepare for what is ahead. Putting a plan in place is essential to avoid making reactive decisions when behaviors are present. Some dementias progress rapidly, while others have a longer trajectory, such as with Alzheimer's disease. Alzheimer's disease can last for twenty years from the time first symptoms appear. This is important to know because a financial plan will need to be in place to ensure money is allocated. Financial planning will be included later in this book. The second reason a specific diagnosis is important is because medications may cause a paradoxical effect, as they are not intended or recommended for use with certain types of dementia. For example, people with Lewy body dementia are highly sensitive to medications provided for behaviors, and the list of medications that are useful is short.

Regardless of the type of dementia, it is always caused by damage to the brain cells. When brain cells are damaged, they are unable to communicate, which leads to the symptoms observed. Depending on the type of dementia and the location in the brain, different characteristics are observed. Studying the brain is a difficult task, particularly since some areas compensate for others when the brain suffers damage.

I attempted to complete a cognitive test to get Margaret's baseline. We started with orientation; she scored a four out of five. She was able to intellectually discuss current events and politics. She enjoyed watching the debates between Donald Trump and Hilary Clinton. I found it fascinating how oriented she was but was significantly impacted by other realms of cognitive function. I attempted to continue cognitive testing, but she became suspicious and refused to continue. I knew she was legally deemed to be an incapacitated adult but never had the ability to fully explore the many facets of her disease.

Margaret spent multiple nights awake, and when she would sleep, it would be limited to a couple of hours. She did not nap during the day. Because of her lack of sleep, I witnessed dramatic shifts of emotions and behaviors. She vacillated from normal, logical conversations to completely erratic and irrational. Part of her difficulty with sleeping was the belief of men coming into her home without permission, and she feared what they would do to her. She stated there is one man who stays outside of her home. When she shines a flashlight, he runs away. There is another man who enters her home. The first time she saw this man was through her blinds in the front bedroom with direct visualization of the front door. She observed him opening the screen door and trying to come through the front door. She told him to go away and he ran. The man eventually had the courage to enter the home. Margaret stated she knew the man was handicap, because his right leg was bent and, as such, he had difficulty walking and running. The man usually did not talk to her but would stare at her. One day he entered her bedroom, put his bent leg on the bed and stated, "Well, are you going to sleep all day?" Margaret stated she wanted to tell him it is none of his business, but she did not have the courage to do so. Another time the man came up behind her, tapped her shoulder and said, "Boo, I'm ISIS," and ran away. After this story came an uncontrollable bout of emotional distress. She screamed how angry she was about ISIS and what they were doing to people. It was as if she was watching these acts of torture as she spoke to me. She would eventually calm down but would cycle through in a couple of hours and scream and cry in terror about ISIS.

Margaret spoke mostly about the man who lived in her attic. It did sound as though the man in the attic was different than the handicap man. She told me he watches her from the attic. He apparently would leave the home and come back. Margaret stated she has no idea how he got into her house because she would lock all the doors. She also put bottles by the front door hoping he would tip them over when he walks in, thus alerting her. She folded paper and put the paper in between doors to determine if the man had used certain doors in the home. One night she picked up folded paper from the closet and showed it to me. She was fearful and stated the man came down from the attic and is probably in the home. She indicated she was not sure if the man was human because she has never observed him entering or leaving through a door. She concluded the man may be walking through the walls. She thought it was possible the man was a demon. I attempted several times to get her out of the home to distract her from these thoughts, but just as I thought she would leave, she told me she was fearful of the man coming in and felt she needed to be there just in case. One night I surprisingly got her to leave her house. I told her we would pick up food and be back quickly. We went to Dunkin' Donuts; she got a sugary coffee drink and donuts. There was a moment of time where she stopped talking about the crisis in her home and truly enjoyed herself. She ate and drank, people-watched, and talked to various customers coming through. It was the first time I saw a smile on her face, which brightened my day.

With Margaret having twenty-four-hour care in her home, I was able to get other perspectives on her behavior. She was intermittently erratic during the day and night hours. She asked one of the caregivers how many times she intended to use the bathroom. She told the caregivers they cannot use the bathroom in her home. There were nights where she laid in bed, crying. She would attempt to nap during the day but would yell and cry about the world changing, stating Donald Trump becoming president is our only hope. She did not want caregivers in her home, but she also was fearful of being alone. She asked the caregivers to check on her every hour when she was resting to make sure the man was not in her room. At times she became angry and would slam doors and kick her dog. The caregivers tried to protect Margaret's dog while she was erratic.

One day, I received a call from Margaret using the caregiver's phone. Margaret stated that she had advised the caregiver, Amy, about the man in the attic, but Amy seemed unphased and not concerned. Amy told Margaret she would not let the man hurt her, and she was not afraid of him. The reason Amy was not afraid is because she knew the man was not real. The man was very real and very scary to Margaret. Margaret stated she did not think she could have Amy in her home because she does not even value her own life. She also stated Amy is a liability because she would not want to be held liable for any harm caused to Amy. While Amy was trying to calm Margaret's fears, she had the opposite effect. I talked to the caregivers about joining Margaret's world, showing concern about the man being present but also bringing calmness to the situation.

To complicate matters, Margaret had six children, who, according to her, had no interest in being in her life. She stated they turned their back on her. She was not surprised because they were all very selfish, according to her. It is difficult in my position because I usually do not get the full back story. With court appointed cases, there is usually conflict within the family, and usually that conflict is a detriment to the health of the ward of the court. I was told

Margaret's children suspected mental illness, but she was never diagnosed. She apparently had erratic behaviors prior to her diagnosis of dementia and was very challenging to have a relationship with.

## MENTAL ILLNESS

Dementia can cause mood and behavioral changes; however, there are situations where behaviors are not due to dementia but rather mental illness. Forty-four percent of adults ages sixty and older will experience a mental disorder in their lifetime. Chronic mental illness (CMI) can co-occur with dementia, which adds another element of complexity. When there is a history of CMI and co-occurring dementia, it is important to evaluate and treat all aspects of the condition.

There are also mental conditions that increase the incidence of dementia. For example, the presence of depression has been shown to have a link with dementia. There are explanations for this, such as a prodromal symptom of dementia, a reaction to cognitive decline, or a separate risk factor for dementia. Dementia itself is known to cause a lack of interest, fatigue, changes in sleeping patterns, and low mood. As mentioned, depression can mimic dementia and should be ruled out as a reversible cause of dementia. More than two-thirds of symptoms of depression and dementia overlap, which makes diagnosis challenging. A recent study indicated dementia can foreshadow a transition from mild cognitive impairment to Alzheimer's disease. The study also found the risk of dementia over the nine-year period of the study was 20 percent greater in individuals who had a low mood at their baseline.

Posttraumatic stress disorder (PTSD) has also shown to have a great impact in people with dementia. In general, older adults with PTSD are inferior to their non-PTSD counterparts in cognitive measures. A study with a sample size of over 180,000 veterans demonstrated that those with PTSD were more than twice as likely to develop dementia. Furthermore, the presence of PTSD with an onset of dementia proves to be challenging in terms of behaviors.

I took care of a gentleman in a hospice inpatient facility with end-stage dementia, who by all accounts was a gentle, kind man. He was a wartime combat veteran who had a diagnosis of PTSD. He experienced violent behaviors and was sent to the inpatient unit to adjust medications to return home safely. He had vivid hallucinations and would strike at anyone close enough to hit. He was delusional, thinking everyone was trying to hurt him. He would scream and disturb others on the unit. In one of his calm moments, he asked for pudding, which I provided. He became angry and threw the entire container at me. With pudding all over me and the floor, I tried my best to calm him down. We had to use medication to calm him down because his agitation was a detriment to his health.

I had another gentleman, who was near the end of his life, spring up from the bed in a fit of anger. He was screaming at me and appeared fearful. I am still shocked he had the energy to act on his anger. With his fists clenched, he walked toward me. Out of fear I tried to get away, to which he chased me down the hall. He went into a room, picked up a chair, and threw it at me. He then grabbed an IV pole and tried to throw it through a window. He went to the front of the facility, picked up a fire extinguisher, and attempted to break the window. As I went to intervene, he put his hands around my neck and was choking me. The moment was so intense, I did not realize I was being choked. Other staff was able to get him off me. I instructed my staff to call 911 as he was a risk to himself and others. The police were able to hold him down so that we could administer an antipsychotic by injection. He did eventually calm down. I am an advocate for calling 911 when situations reach a level where there is an imminent risk. Sometimes it is necessary.

When a person with dementia has a mental illness, it is important to engage the services of a psychiatrist experienced in dementia, who can work closely with the neurologist. The need for inpatient psychiatric care may be needed at some point in the disease process. It is imperative to remember, the behaviors are a result of damage to the brain and the person does not have control over their behaviors. A person who is paranoid or delusional and who cannot think logically is not able to enter your world.

I have also cared for clients who do not have dementia or a cognitive impairment at their baseline but who exhibit profound cognitive abnormalities when mental illness is not managed. I cared for a woman who scored high on cognitive tests and functioned very well. When she had manic episodes, she behaved like someone with middle-stage dementia, in addition to erratic behaviors. When she came out of her manic episodes, she remembered very little of what occurred and was shocked by some of her behaviors.

I suspect Margaret's children were correct about mental illness. The fact that she was estranged from all her children demonstrates some long-standing family difficulties. Having a specific dementia diagnosis would have been helpful to distinguish between mental illness and dementia-related behaviors. Due to Margaret's intense paranoia and the overall effect on her life, Margaret was transitioned into a mental-health facility to stabilize her condition. Managing her behaviors in the home environment was not possible as she was resistant to taking medication, and the variations in her mood were not healthy for her overall quality of life. Margaret experienced a rapid decline in her health and was later placed into a long-term care facility once she was stabilized. Margaret died peacefully shortly after her move to a facility. I chose to remember the smiling woman eating a donut and drinking coffee in the late afternoon. There was a glimpse of a happy and fun woman when she let her guard down a little.

# Chapter 4:
# Managing Behaviors

Our greatest glory is not in never falling,
but in rising every time we fall.

—Confucius

Behavioral and psychological abnormalities are common at some point in the dementia trajectory. Symptoms can include anxiety, depression, agitation, physical and verbal aggression, and sleep disturbance. As many as 90 percent of people with dementia suffer from behavioral abnormalities. For some people, behavioral disturbance occurs infrequently or in response to evident triggers that would cause psychological distress in anyone. Some people with dementia will exhibit behaviors during a specific phase of their dementia and behaviors dissipate later in the disease. Some people with dementia experience behavioral disturbance throughout the course of the disease, with high intensity at certain points of the disease process. With that said, it is more likely than not the person you are caring for will display behaviors at some point. Before providing information on managing behaviors, I would like to share a method of understanding the mind of a person with dementia.

The *theory of retrogenesis*, which literally means back to birth, was developed by Dr. Barry Reisberg, who has researched cognitive impairment and subsequently published numerous articles over the past thirty-five years. Although this theory is specific to Alzheimer's disease, the implications can be useful for other types of dementia. Dr. Reisberg hypothesizes the brain unravels in the reverse order of the brain's development from birth.

There are pivotal moments after birth to about one-and-a-half years of age that show normal cognitive function. The first of these is the ability to smile. As a newborn continues to grow, we expect the ability to hold the head up, to roll over, to sit up unassisted, to crawl, and eventually to walk. The beginning of vocabulary is also a positive indicator of cognitive structuring. As a toddler, ages two to four, there are various independent tasks that start to emerge. One of which is the ability to use the bathroom. This is a two-part process. First, the act of recognizing the need to urinate or defecate and doing so in the toilet. And second, the process of knowing the mechanics of toileting, such as flushing the toilet and washing hands. A toddler will build on their vocabulary and learn how to dress themselves, which is also a two-part process. The first part is the act of dressing, such as using a zipper or buttoning a shirt. The second part is the ability to dress appropriately, such as the order clothing is put on and choosing clothing suitable to the weather.

Activities of daily living, such as feeding oneself, brushing teeth, and performing grooming independently, will begin to be an autonomous activity. From toddler to adolescence, ages five to eleven, a child becomes fully independent with activities of daily living, dressing appropriately, speaking a wider vocabulary, engaging in social activity, and learning about money. As children continue to grow, they learn to drive, gain employment, manage bills, live independently, and perhaps start a family of their own.

The theory of retrogenesis postulates a person with Alzheimer's disease will experience regression of the same cognitive indicators in the reverse order, which is proportionate with the degradation of the brain. Before proceeding, I want to emphasize these classifications are not to imply a person with Alzheimer's disease, or any form of dementia, is childlike or to be treated like a child. A person with dementia deserves respect and to be treated with compassion and understanding. This theory has helped me frame my thinking around the most respectful approach to care for someone with dementia.

An individual with early Alzheimer's disease may still be working and running a household but is having more difficulty doing so. There may be lapses in memory requiring frequent reminders or misplacement of commonly used items. You may notice difficulty in finding words, in managing money, with directions while driving, and with social interaction. An individual with early Alzheimer's disease is cognitively functioning in the five- to eleven-year-old age range. As the disease progresses into the middle stage, the cognitive advancements seen from the ages of two to four are now difficult. A person in the middle stage of Alzheimer's disease has difficulty getting dressed, is losing vocabulary, and having difficulty ambulating. Falls become more frequent during this stage. Urinary and bowel control may be impacted, which is the same two-part process in reverse. Initially, the mechanics of toileting are affected, so the person with Alzheimer's disease may forget the need to pull pants up or to wash their hands. The second action of dressing is also impacted, so the person may put their bra over their shirt or wear snow boots in the summer. Cognitively speaking, a person in the middle stage of Alzheimer's disease is functioning at the level of a two- to four-year-old.

The late stage of Alzheimer's is comparable to infancy to one-and-a-half years old in cognitive capability. A person with late-stage Alzheimer's will forget how to walk and eventually stop walking altogether. Vocabulary is lost until there are only a few words or a string of words that do not belong together; speech may even be unintelligible or rarely occurring. The first stage of dressing and toileting are severely impacted. Continence is eventually lost, and the person with Alzheimer's needs incontinence care. In the very last stage, the ability to sit up unassisted, hold one's head up, and smile is gone. Additionally, swallowing is altered and the risk for aspiration is high. The creator of the theory of retrogenesis, Dr. Barry Reisberg, also developed the Functional Assessment Staging (FAST) scale, which was mentioned previously as a tool commonly used by hospice organizations to assist with determining eligibility. The FAST scale is useful when dementia is more advanced and traditional means of testing cognition is no longer useful. The scale goes from stage 1 (normal adult) to 7E (end-stage Alzheimer's). On that scale, 7E is the loss of the ability to smile, which, as mentioned, was the first indicator of cognitive development.

What is incredibly useful with this theory is the ability to better understand why a person with dementia is acting a certain way and to develop strategies to best manage behaviors. Keeping the theory in mind, what techniques would you use with an eleven-year-old or a three-year-old or even an infant? Imagine an infant is crying and cannot be consoled. What would you do? I would imagine you would investigate further to determine why the infant is crying. The infant may be hungry and need a diaper changed. An infant is going to communicate with you the only way they know how. A person with dementia can only communicate the way they know how, such as through crying or screaming. It is your role to determine what is being communicated and to provide the care that is needed.

I think middle-stage-dementia behaviors are the most difficult to understand and care for. There are many times I have witnessed other health-care professionals use medication to calm this behavior, which is appropriate at times, but should not be the first response. If your three-year-old were kicking and screaming, you may choose to allow them to get it out of their system or there could be something wrong that needs further investigating. People with dementia need the tender care and compassion we would provide to our own child.

I was recently with a client in the ER, which is traumatic for someone with dementia. The physician ordered a urinalysis to determine if she had a UTI. There were two nurses who were attempting to get urine through a catheter. My client was scared and upset. Imagine you are in a strange place and do not understand what is happening and strangers are trying to pull down your pants. I know I would fight back, which is what she did. One of the nurses yelled, "You need to let us do what we need to do to take care of you." I was able to intervene. I moved directly in her view and made eye contact. I held her hand and gently talked her through what was happening. She was not trying to be difficult; she was terrified.

You may have already experienced behavioral disturbance in caring for someone with dementia and felt frightened or felt like you would not be able to provide ongoing care. You may be worried about behaviors in the future and want tools to get through those difficult moments. In managing behaviors, I always start with non-pharmacological treatment, and if necessary, will advocate for medication. Medication should not be for convenience; it should be used to improve the quality of life for someone with dementia. I am going to provide tips for challenging behaviors, but know that not all these tactics work on everyone. You may need to adjust the approach to best suit the needs of the person you are caring for. Before reviewing common behaviors, I want to present a tactic known as therapeutic fibbing, which is a tactic that can be used for any behavior. It is useful to understand this tactic before reviewing common behaviors because it can be used in addition to the tactics I provide in each section.

## THERAPEUTIC FIBBING

Honesty is not always the best policy when having a conversation with a person with dementia. Honesty forces the person with dementia to enter your reality when we should be stepping into the reality of the person with dementia. I have consulted with families that feel guilty about lying to their loved one, but a therapeutic fib is a compassionate approach when not used to be malicious or unnecessarily misleading. I think of a therapeutic fib as a gateway to entering the reality of the person with dementia. There is certainly a time for honesty in communicating with a person with dementia. You will have to distinguish between when an honest approach is the most compassionate method and when therapeutic fibbing is necessary to promote comfort and peace.

One example I run into commonly is when a person with dementia says, "I need to get ready for work." The honest approach would entail telling the person they are retired and do not need to worry about getting ready for work. This will likely cause frustration, confusion, and possibly anger.

The therapeutic approach would be to validate the statement and offer a distraction, such as eating breakfast before getting ready. When distracted, the person with dementia will forget they indicated that they need to get ready for work. The statement may be repeated, but it would be most compassionate to validate and distract. This could also entail going for a ride in the car and going somewhere your loved one enjoys.

Another common comment I hear is, "Have you seen my husband?" The honest approach would be to tell the person with dementia their loved one is dead. The person with dementia will grieve the death all over again and feel upset they forgot their spouse is dead. The therapeutic approach would be to state their husband ran to the store. I had a client who initially knew her husband had died, but after physical and mental abuse at the hands of her son, she completely forgot her husband died. She would ask where he was or make comments indicating he was on his way to pick her up. Her abusive son stated she should be confronted with honesty so she can come to terms with the reality. Doing so would be very upsetting for her, and because she has dementia, she would forget. Telling her repeatedly that her husband is dead would not help her come to terms with reality and would only traumatize her every time she was told the truth.

Some therapeutic fibs can be more challenging. I had a client who had a change in her health and needed to go to a skilled nursing facility until she was stable to go back to her assisted living apartment. She had a private caregiver with her because she was forgetful and confused and became emotionally distraught when she did not understand what was happening. I witnessed her go to the nurse's station to ask where she was. The staff would tell her she is in a nursing facility. She would ask why. They would tell her she came from the hospital and her doctor ordered physical therapy. She stated she had not been to the hospital and demanded to know what doctor ordered therapy. When told the doctor's name, she stated she did not know who that person was, and she became agitated and angry. I talked to the staff about a better approach to avoid causing undue stress and anxiety, but it usually fell on deaf ears. After the staff would upset her, I would get her back to her room. She stated she needed to leave right away. I told her she needed to stay the night because there is some maintenance work being done in her apartment. She asked for details, so I told her there was water leakage and her floor was being replaced. She was content with staying the night. She, of course, would not remember this the next day. One day she told me she bought a plane ticket to go home to Ohio. She was adamant about going to the airport. I faked a call and told her the flight was delayed because of snow. I told her we would need to stay the night in what she thought was a hotel and hopefully we can fly out tomorrow. These strategies kept her calm and improved her quality of life.

I use therapeutic fibbing on many occasions. There are times the person with dementia does not believe what I am saying and may even become agitated. I generally provide a distraction and use a different approach for the therapeutic fib once the memory of the previous fib is gone. Knowing a person's story is helpful in coming up with therapeutic fibs, as you can incorporate their past life into their new, distorted reality.

## AGITATION

Agitation is a common occurrence with dementia and is frightening when behaviors turn aggressive. Symptoms of agitation include emotional outbursts, delusions, hallucinations, pacing/wandering, frequent movement, and use of threatening language. Agitation can be the result of many causes:

- Medical conditions and medication side effects should be assessed first. One major medical cause of agitation is infections. In those who are elderly with dementia, agitation is usually the first symptom. Infections may also present with delirium, which is an abrupt disturbance in mentation, causing severe confusion and, potentially, hallucinations. Any acute change should be evaluated by a physician immediately. Other medical conditions should also be considered. Often, medical conditions in people with dementia are overlooked, as professionals and others attribute symptoms mainly to dementia. Medication side effects can cause a range of cognitive and mental side effects. If a new medication has been started or a medication dosage has been changed, a medication side effect should be considered.

- Subjective symptoms, such as pain, constipation, full bladder, hunger, feeling too hot or too cold, and tight clothing.
- Changes in environment, such as moving to a new location, changing of furniture, or even changes in the people who are providing care.
- Fear, which can be real or imagined. Fear can be amplified by poor sight or poor lighting, leading to visual perception of items or people that are not there. Delusions and hallucinations can also be fearful.
- Fatigue, which causes agitation in most people. Imagine your entire world is confusing and you are also tired.

If possible, prevent agitation from occurring. This may be accomplished by ensuring a calm environment, using soothing rituals, removing triggers, using adequate lighting, having vision checked, promoting daytime activities, allowing for periods of rest, and providing a routine.

When caring for someone with dementia, it is important to remember the person is living in a world that no longer makes sense. We cannot expect the person to enter our world. As the caregiver or loved one, we must step inside their world and meet the person where they are in their disease. When confronted with agitation, it is our respon-sibility to put on a detective hat and attempt to understand why agitation is occurring. When the person you are caring for becomes agitated, there are some tactics that may be beneficial. Approaches to manage agitation include the following:

- Determine the cause of agitation and remove bar-riers causing distress. This should always be the first step. Pain is a common cause of agitation with dementia. Many times, I have seen an elderly person with dementia transferred into a chair in a swift manner, which likely causes pain due to arthritis and other aging factors. As a response, the patient may strike out or scream. Imagine you are experiencing pain and want someone to stop what they are doing that is causing pain, but you cannot put into words how you feel. You may strike or scream. Consider repositioning, using more pillows, or transferring slowly. Track bowel movements to make sure constipation is not an issue. If the person you are caring for can communicate on some level, ask what is bothering them. Your approach should be gentle and caring. If you have identified agita-tion is not due to a physical issue or discomfort, you can try other approaches. You may use the other approaches in conjunction with correcting the issue causing agitation.

- Provide redirection. A person with dementia can usually concentrate on one topic or event at a time. If agitation is occurring and you can distract to another activity, the agitation may dissipate as the brain is shifting focus toward another activity. Ideas for redirection include going for a walk, looking at pictures, working on a puzzle together, or providing a snack.

- Provide reassurance. Ensure the person with dementia knows that they are safe and that you will stay with them. Ask the person if you can help them, and let them know you are sorry for the way they feel.

- Limit stimulation. An overstimulated environment can be overwhelming and lead to agitation. If there are noises coming from different areas, try to reduce noises to one source. If there are many people in the home, try to limit the amount of people near the person you are caring for. I have witnessed clients who do well with one person but become agitated when there are two or more people in their line of sight.

- Do not argue or try to reason. Thinking back to the theory of retrogenesis, you would not argue or reason with a child who has a cognitive functioning level of a two-year-old. If you have tried to do that before, you probably know you will never win that fight. Being right is not worth the consequences that will ensue.

- If agitation turns into physical aggression, walk away. You will also need to remove objects that can be used as a weapon. Give the person space to calm down, approach slowly from the front, and use eye contact. If your physical safety is in jeopardy, it is appropriate to call 911. I had a client whose agitation was hastened by loud noises and being startled. One of the nurses came into his room when he was sleeping, startled him, and she then started to speak very loudly. My client became enraged, got out of bed, grabbed the blood pressure machine, and threw it at her. He was screaming and using profanity. His wife came to visit him when this was occurring, and he punched her in the face. He was a calm and gentle man, and this behavior was unusual for him. Emergency services were contacted as he was at risk of physically hurting others around him.
- If agitation and/or aggression is occurring despite interventions, you should consult with a medical professional. Although medications should be used as a last resort, there are some people with dementia that require stabilizing medication. Your physician can help determine if the use of medication is appropriate.

## EATING

Challenges with eating occur on both sides of the spectrum. With dementia, the area of the brain that controls hunger (hypothalamus) is damaged. This is not true with all dementias; however, with continued disease progression, all areas of the brain can become affected. Earlier in the disease process, a person with dementia may have increased hunger and eat more than their metabolic needs. This is partially due to forgetfulness. If a person with dementia does not remember eating, she may assume it is time to eat.

Many client families are concerned about weight gain during this part of the disease. Weight gain is not a negative aspect in earlier phases unless other medical conditions are impacted by weight gain. Later in the disease process, the hypothalamus changes and appetite decreases. Putting on weight earlier in the disease process allows the person with dementia to have a buffer when appetite decreases, and weight loss accelerates. On the other side of the spectrum, many client families are concerned that they cannot get their loved one to eat healthy meals or that intake is significantly decreased. It is important to have the physician evaluate all medications to ensure medications are not causing nausea or a decreased appetite. In fact, some medications for dementia can cause nausea and impact appetite, even if the medication is not new to the person with dementia.

Distractions during mealtime should be kept to a minimum. The environment should be calm and inviting. Providing only the utensils needed for the meal decreases confusion. There should be different color contrasts between the plate and the placemat because of visual perception changes, as mentioned previously. It is recommended to serve larger meals in the morning or afternoon and encourage snacking during the day. High-caloric shakes can assist in supplementing nutrients. A shake can be made with ingredients your loved one enjoys, such as ice cream or fruit. Adding protein powder is a bonus.

An often-overlooked cause of decreased appetite is poor oral health and dental issues. Loose dentures may cause pain and even sores in the mouth, which would naturally decrease intake. Additionally, a dry mouth can make eating difficult or change the way food tastes. Other oral issues, such as infected teeth, also cause pain and impact the ability to eat. When bacteria grow in the mouth, the taste of foods can be affected, thus affecting appetite. Also, people who are on antibiotics have an increased risk of thrush, which is a fungal infection in the mouth. This causes changes in taste and oral pain.

While on the subject of oral health, I recommend continuation of dental appointments, especially with dementia. People with dementia may not brush their teeth as well as they should and tend to have more dental issues. I have clients who see the dentist every three months for a deep cleaning to ensure adequate oral health. Decreased oral hygiene is also an indicator of cognitive impairment if dementia has not been suspected previously. In my personal life, I had not seen my grandfather for several years. When I visited with him, I noticed his bottom teeth were rotting. I was surprised by this as he was always a well-kept person. I suspected cognitive impairment because of my background, but I also thought he was lacking in hygiene due to the stress of my grandmother's death. I did find out several months later that my grandfather did, in fact, have dementia.

Many clients' family members have commented that their loved one only wants to eat sweets and that they are concerned about their nutritional level. A sweet tooth occurs commonly in the elderly. This is partially due to decreased taste buds and other foods lacking taste. With dementia, the part of the brain that controls cravings can be altered and the person with dementia may lack restraint. You can use a sweet tooth to your advantage. Try sprinkling some sugar or chocolate syrup over food. I know it sounds disgusting, but a person with dementia will eat food based on taste without perceiving what they are eating. I have heard of people putting chocolate syrup over broccoli. It is like a compromise the person with dementia is not aware of. If diabetes is an issue, use an artificial sweetener. This should be used with caution as some artificial sweeteners have health consequences.

Maintaining adequate fluid intake is also challenging. Dehydration can cause the skin to be more prone to breakdown, increase the risk of urinary tract infections, increase confusion, and lead to constipation. The person with dementia usually does not have an awareness of thirst and needs you to assist in staying hydrated. I recommend offering fluids every hour, because generally only sips are taken. Fluids do not have to be water, although some fluids should be water. I have one client who tells me she is not thirsty when offered fluids, so I either drink fluids with her or I ask her to taste the fluid I am giving her.

## INCONTINENCE

In general, as a person ages, physical changes can cause incontinence, which is the loss of bowel or bladder control. With a diagnosis of dementia, it is important to rule out medical conditions that cause incontinence. In the earlier states of most dementias, incontinence is usually not present, but as the disease advances, incontinence is an expected deficit. Although, one type of dementia, normal pressure hydrocephalus (NPH), presents with urinary incontinence along with difficulty walking and cognitive impairment. Initially, incontinence may occur due to the failure to get to the bathroom in time or difficulty in removing clothing while in the bathroom. There are tactics to lengthen the ability to control continence.

For urinary incontinence, try keeping a record of incontinence episodes. The log can assist in developing a toileting schedule according to your loved one's needs. Scheduled toileting is recommended, which entails taking the person you are caring for to the toilet every two to four hours. Make scheduling toileting part of the daily routine. Watch for cues, such as facial expression, that indicate the need to use the bathroom. Provide clothing that is easy to remove and put back on. At some point, the person you are caring for may forget where the bathroom is. You may recall from chapter two that Shirley could not remember where the bathroom was and was found urinating in the closet. I have also witnessed people with dementia urinating in trash cans or potted plants. This is very common as the disease progresses. A sign that reads toilet with a picture of a toilet on or by the door is helpful and promotes dignity.

A good habit to implement is to provide a small cup of water after each restroom trip to promote hydration. One of the most important factors regarding bowel management is adequate fluid intake. Additionally, activity assists in stimulating the bowels. To assist with fluid intake, provide foods that have a high-water content. Incorporating fiber into the diet is also helpful. As the disease progresses, the person with dementia may lose the instinct to push. Ensure medications are not causing constipation. Even supplements, such as calcium and iron, can cause constipation. Constipation can cause a loss of appetite and discomfort. If the bowels are not moving, the risk for impaction is present. I have cared for clients with dementia who require intermittent disimpaction, which is removal of stool manually, because the urge to push is not present. Keep in mind, the presence of loose stools may be an indication of constipation, because stool will squeeze around the impaction and give the appearance of diarrhea. There are many medications that assist with constipation and may be needed on a consistent basis.

If diarrhea is occurring, the cause should be evaluated. I have taken care of many people who are eating spoiled and expired food from their refrigerator and pantry, and once the refrigerator and pantry are cleaned, the diarrhea goes away. Some medications can cause diarrhea. If diarrhea persists for no apparent reason, the physician needs to be consulted to ensure there is not a medical cause for the diarrhea.

With incontinence comes the need to ensure adequate skin care. At some point, you may need to take over personal care after using the bathroom. The goal is to keep the person you are caring for as clean and dry as possible. Pull-up briefs can be helpful, and some people use a pad inside of the brief for extra protection. If using a brief, the brief needs to be checked every couple of hours. Lack of proper continence care can lead to skin breakdown and infections.

## BATHING

One of the biggest challenges I am consulted on regards bathing. I have heard many stories about failed attempts at bathing and can understand the stress it can cause. Fortunately, there are some tactics that may be useful. In earlier stages of dementia, a person may continue their normal bathing routine. A person with dementia may change their routines due to forgetfulness and unawareness of their appearance. Consider how depression could be an additional factor when hygiene has changed in the person you are caring for. Although bathing challenges do not occur with everyone with dementia, it is a common issue faced by caregivers. The middle stage of dementia seems to present the most challenges. Failure to maintain hygiene may be the first indication of dementia for some people.

During the cognitive level associated with the middle stage of dementia, the bathing experience is much different, and it requires us to enter the world of the person we are caring for. Previously we discussed changes in visual acuity with dementia: persons with dementia have a lens of vision that is straight ahead—meaning not up, down, or peripheral. Running water from a shower head that cannot be seen can be scary. The person with dementia may not understand where the water is coming from and why water is hitting their head. Additionally, the hypothalamus, which affects appetite, also affects the ability to regulate body temperature. When the hypothalamus is affected, a person with dementia generally feels cold. You may have noticed the person you are caring for complaining of being cold when you feel warm.

Ensure the bathing area is suitable to the needs of the person you are caring for. A shower chair is recommended, as well as non-slip mats, grab bars, and a removeable shower head.

Prior to the bathing experience, prepare the bathing area to ensure the temperature is warm and comfortable for the person you are caring for. Keep in mind, this may not be a comfortable temperature for you. Run the water ahead of time to make sure the water is warm. Place all items needed for the shower and after the shower nearby. When bringing your loved one into the bathroom, remember undressing may feel uncomfortable and embarrassing. Promote dignity by providing reassurance. You can also hold up a towel while your loved one undresses to provide privacy. I generally run warm water on the shower chair to warm it up and then give the removeable shower head to the person to allow as much independence as possible.

Whenever you are providing additional assistance, always tell the person what you are going to do to help. If there is a fear of water, you can use a hand towel to get the hair wet and to remove shampoo and conditioner. Try to make the bathing experience as enjoyable as possible. You can massage their back, use pleasant aromas, or any other luxury that you know your loved one enjoys. After the shower, massage lotion into the skin, if this is not an irritant. Put a warm robe on after the shower. After the shower, doing their hair or painting nails adds to the experience.

Lastly, do not force the issue. If the person tells you no, do not argue. The only perceived benefit of memory loss is that you can reapproach the person in five minutes and try again. Maybe use a different approach the next time. A sweet treat may entice your loved one to bathe.

Another common bathing struggle occurs when the person with dementia believes they already showered and exert their independence by expressing offense in the suggestion of bathing. I have a client with a sense of smell that is non-existent, so she does not have an awareness of her body odor. She also wears the same robe every day. If bathing is suggested, she snaps back, stating she showers every morning and does not need to be told when to shower. We try to find activities out of the home, which leads her to shower and get dressed. The robe is put in the wash when she is not aware. We are constantly searching for ways to get her to shower without offending her and causing agitation. There can be a very fine balance, and even as a health-care professional, I find the bathing battle to be particularly challenging.

It is important to remember a shower is not necessary every day. At a certain age, daily showers can dry out the skin and cause discomfort. Most older people shower about three times a week. What I call a bird bath can be done in between showers or even in lieu of a shower if the person is not agreeable to a shower. By using a warm washcloth, areas of the body can be cleaned. A non-rinse cleanser is also helpful in between showers. There are also non-rinse shampoos and shower caps that contain a non-rinse shampoo that can be used if washing hair is an issue.

## DRESSING

As the disease progresses and the brain forgets how to do simple tasks, dressing inappropriately will occur. Initially, you may notice the sequence of clothing is not correct, such as underwear outside the clothing, as well as a difficulty matching clothes and dressing for the season. Some cognitive examinations ask what the current season is. Most clients guess incorrectly, by answering summer when it is winter, for example, which makes dressing appropriately difficult. Further damage to the brain leads to inability to know how to put clothing on and how to button a shirt.

As with anything related to dementia, you want to make the selection of clothing as simple as possible. Instead of asking, "What do you want to wear?" you can ask, "Do you want to wear the black shirt or the blue shirt?" It is also helpful to organize the process by which you lay out the clothing in the order it needs to be put on, to minimize distractions and to follow a routine for dressing.

Dressing will become a step-by-step process. Instead of directing your loved one to put on a shirt, you will have to say, "Put your arm through this sleeve, put your other arm through this sleeve, put your head through the shirt." This can be difficult at first, because these actions are automatic for us, but for the person with dementia, one instruction at a time is needed. Assisting with dressing requires patience. Because you are going through each step, you will notice it takes at least twice the amount of time to get dressed.

One of the biggest concerns expressed by families is that the same clothing has been worn every day and that their loved one appears dirty. It is helpful to be flexible and allow the person you are caring for to wear an outfit for two days or have duplicates of outfits so you can rotate washing. Most people with dementia have a few outfits they prefer to wear, and their preference is usually the most comfortable clothing in their closet. Pants that pull up and do not have a button or zipper are helpful. This is also helpful when the person with dementia starts to have incontinence, as the time it takes to pull the pants down is reduced. Shoes should be slip-on or Velcro strapped. Ensure the tread on shoes provides safety.

## SLEEPING

Many older adults have difficulty sleeping, but people with dementia tend to have even more sleep issues. This becomes challenging for the caregiver who is awake during the day and has a loved one up at night. The most common sleep issue with dementia is decreased hours of sleep in the middle stages and increased sleep in the advanced stages. Causes of decreased sleep may be due to a medical cause, anxiety, or overstimulation. There is also a phenomenon known as sundowning, which generally occurs later in the day, and presents with increased confusion, agitation, paranoia, and aggression. Sundowning can occur if there is more activity in the environment later in the day and is the result of increased fatigue due to the sun going down, changes in circadian rhythm, or reduced lighting causing shadows.

I have experienced sundowning with persons with dementia many times in my career, some occurrences being minor and other occurrences being harmful. For example, when I was out with my client, we decided to get something to eat around 4:00 p.m. Although memory impairment was evident, she seemed oriented to herself and the place. Almost as though someone turned off a switch, she looked at me and asked, "How long have you been in Palm Springs?" I was taken aback initially and had to tap into my experience to respond in a respectful manner. I entered her world and answered her question as though we were dining in Palm Springs.

The worst episode of sundowning I have witnessed was when I was a hospice nurse. My patient was newly on hospice for dementia and other complicating medical conditions. She was living with her husband at home, where her daughter stopped by often to check on them. I received a call from the husband in a panic, asking me to come over immediately. I asked questions to understand what was occurring. The husband told me his wife thinks he is her pimp and got ahold of a knife. His daughter came over and was able to get her to put down the knife before the police had to be called. I made a visit after it was safe to enter. I learned my patient had sundowning behaviors frequently and her delusions usually involved her husband being a stranger to her. She would wake up in the middle of the night and panic when she woke up next to the stranger, who was her husband. There were times she thought her husband was a pimp. She even stated the pimp in her home opens the window at night to let men in for services. She was terrified, and her husband was distressed. My patient did require medications to help with delusions and paranoia in the evening hours, which greatly improved her and her husband's quality of life. Although sundowning behaviors generally occur later in the day, there are some people with dementia that sundown earlier in the day.

Another common sleeping behavior is sleep deprivation. For those of you caring for someone with dementia at home, this can prove to be especially challenging. I have cared for clients who are awake for two to three days at a time. When they do sleep, it is usually for an entire day. Recall Margaret from chapter three: her intense fear and paranoia caused her to stay awake for days at a time. While fear and paranoia can cause someone with dementia to stay awake, other factors may also be present. For example, a person with dementia who used to work nights may have a sense of comfort in being awake at night. These people may also think they need to go to work and become anxious if they cannot figure out how to get to work. I have also cared for clients who woke up as early as 3:00 a.m. to get ready for work, yet no longer working and with dementia, they would sleep briefly and were still programmed to wake up at 3:00 a.m. Having patient history clarifies why this behavior is occurring.

To promote better sleeping patterns, you should consult with the physician to determine if there is a medical cause for the behavior. Some conditions can cause difficulty with sleep, and as such, it should not be automatically assumed dementia is causing the disturbance. It is also worthwhile to rule out sleep apnea, as this can affect sleep and reduce oxygenation to the brain. Additionally, medication can be the cause. All medications should be evaluated for side effects. Even without sleep behaviors, people with dementia do best when there is a routine.

Having consistent times for eating, activities, and other events helps promote overall stability in a person with dementia. Physical activity during the day may assist in feeling tired later in the day. Physical activity can be as simple as going for a walk. If this is a part of the daily routine, even better. The nighttime hours should be calm and peaceful. Think of what makes the person you are caring for feel relaxed. Stimulants, such as caffeine, should be minimal during the day and not used at night. Also, too many fluids in the evening hours increases the chance of waking up to urinate at night. It is recommended to limit daytime napping, although as the disease progresses, naps may be a necessity. Discouraging napping for some people can increase agitation and could lead to sleeping behaviors. It may be worth considering melatonin to improve sleep. Melatonin is a natural supplement and is generally safe to use with dementia. I am leery of prescription-sleeping medication, as there are many side effects and may not assist with the issue. Lastly, ensure proper light in the evening hours. I have a client who starts to sundown when the sun is coming down. We have started to routinely turn on lights around the house before it gets dark outside to counter the behavior. It generally prevents sundowning behavior.

There may be some simple adjustments that can be made to assist sleeping behaviors, while some people with dementia will continue unusual sleeping behaviors despite all efforts. Sometimes it makes more sense to allow the person with dementia to have altered sleeping arrangements. For example, for the person who worked nights all their life, changing the sleep schedule may not be feasible. You may need to bring someone in at night if the alteration in sleep is affecting your ability to be a caregiver during the day.

## REPETITIVE BEHAVIORS

A person with dementia may ask the same question multiple times, with little time between each question. This can be frustrating at a certain point. I had a client who would ask the date about twenty times before moving to another question that was repeated about twenty times. I would answer the question the same as though it was the first time it was asked to preserve dignity, but eventually I did have to attempt to stop the behavior.

The best counter for repetitive behaviors is to provide a distraction. The client I mentioned loved solving other people's problems. I would make up a life problem, and she would give advice about what I should do. I would listen and comment on how helpful she was. This would stop the line of questioning because she was engaged in helping me. Other ideas for distraction include going for a walk, playing music, and working on a puzzle, or you can ignore the behavior.

I heard a story of a gentleman who would take his mother to the store weekly. He became aggravated by her asking where they were going the entire drive, so he wrote a note, placed it on her lap, and would direct her to read the note when she would ask where they were going. The other tactic to stop repetitive behaviors is to engage the person with dementia in a repetitive activity. For example, put towels in a laundry basket and ask your loved one to fold them. Once done, you can express appreciation for the help, unfold the towels and bring them back to be folded. You could also get a set of nuts and bolts and ask your loved one to sort and organize them or get different sized PVC pipes and allow your loved one to put them together. The activity should coincide with your loved one's past. For example, a person who was a secretary may do well folding papers, putting them in envelopes, and organizing. If your loved one is artistic, set up an easel and allow them to paint, or work on art crafts together. Many family members will have their loved one help around the house, under supervision. Aiding with tasks gives the person with dementia a sense of accomplishment and helps them feel useful.

## WANDERING

Wandering is a challenging behavior that usually occurs in the middle stage of dementia; however, it can occur at any stage of the disease. According to the Alzheimer's Association (2015), 60 percent of people with dementia will wander at some point over the course of their disease. As with any behavior, the cause of wandering must be evaluated. People with dementia wander for a variety of reasons:

- **Confusion.** Wandering is often related to a lack of awareness to time and place, as well as to a difficulty recognizing people and objects. The person with dementia may wander to explore answers about their confusing world. Some people with dementia do not recognize their environment and conclude they are not home. They may ask or demand to go home. This scenario puts a person with dementia at a very high risk of wandering. Additionally, if a person with dementia woke up in what seems to be a strange place, they may try to escape out of fear of the unknown.
- **Agitation.** As mentioned previously, agitation can be caused by many factors, which should be investigated and managed as best as possible.
- **Medication.** If wandering is a new behavior that occurred after starting a new medication or changing the dosage of an existing medication, consider the

medication as the cause of the new behavior. This is true for any alteration after a change in medication.

I have met with many families of people with dementia and provided recommendations regarding safety, which includes wandering behaviors. Many times a family member has said, "Well, she hasn't wandered yet." Do not wait for the "yet" before taking actions to prevent wandering. Techniques to manage wandering behaviors include the following:

- **Ensure all needs are met.** If the behavior is due to a factor you can control, address what is causing discomfort. Once the issue is resolved, wandering behaviors may cease.
- **Provide reassurance.** Just as you would reassure when agitation is present, it is important to reassure a person with wandering behaviors that they are safe, and you are there to help. If the behaviors are due to wanting to go home, listen to their words, validate their feelings, explore the meaning in their words, and reassure. A therapeutic fib can go a long way in these situations. For example, if the person with dementia states they want to go home, you can validate your understanding of their desire to go home and ask them to stay one more night with you. I had a client who routinely stated she was going home the next day and needed to pack. The staff at the assisted living would tell her she is home and there is no need to pack. This increased

her agitation. Instead, I asked the staff to acknowledge her need to pack to go home tomorrow, ensure she feels safe for the night, and let her pack if it helps with her anxiety. She did not recognize her apartment at night and was fearful. Allowing her to stay in her reality instead of forcing the staff's reality alleviated her anxiety and fear.

- **Promote activity.** Keeping the person with dementia busy with a task interrupts the behavior, so include activities such as exercising and assisting around the home.

- **Secure the home.** Even if wandering has never been an issue. Due to changes in peripheral vision, a person with dementia generally does not look up or down. As such, locks can be placed high or low so that they are not seen. Additionally, vision changes with dementia causes altered perception. A dark area may appear to be a hole. I notice this when I am out with a client and there are different colors on the ground. In darker areas, the person with dementia usually picks their feet up higher and gently puts their feet down as they cannot perceive the depth with changing colors. As such, you could place a dark rug by the door, which would appear to be a hole. As always, this should be done with caution, as rugs increase fall risk. Another technique is to paint the door and door knob the same color of the wall. A person with dementia will not realize there is a door there. I have seen many memory-care units that have the door painted to blend in with the wall. One memory-care unit painted the door to look like a bookcase. Another one painted a tree that started on the wall, covered the door, and extended to the wall on the other side of the door.

- **Inform your neighbors.** Let your neighbors know you are caring for a person with dementia. Ask neighbors to call if they see the person you are caring for outside alone. Obviously if wandering does occur, you need to search immediately. Ninety-four percent of people with dementia that wander are found within a mile and a half of where they disappeared from. Search the perimeter of the location of where your loved one went missing. Additionally, most people who wander will wander in the direction of their dominant hand.

- **Consider a GPS device.** There are several options. I recommend going to the Alzheimer's Association website and searching devices or The Alzheimer's Store for devices and a variety of products geared for caring for a person with dementia.

## Suspicious Behavior

With the loss of memory and living in a confusing world, a person with dementia may become suspicious. This can present with your loved one being suspicious of you or others and accusations of theft. When this happens, it is important to remember this behavior is normal, not a reflection of something you did wrong. Listen to the cause of suspicious behavior and then reassure the person you are caring for that you will help and that you care about their distress. Arguing, explaining, or convincing will prove to be fruitless and will cause increased agitation and paranoia. Redirection can be helpful if possible. I have experienced instances where the person with dementia is so focused on the source of their suspiciousness that redirection is not possible. Generally, when an item is missing, it is because the person with dementia has hidden the object and does not remember where it was placed. Having duplicates of some items can be helpful, such as two of the same wallet or purse.

Some people with dementia have recurring suspicious behavior that impacts their daily life. When the overall quality of life is affected by this, or any behavior, it is worth considering a low dose of a medication to assist. Documenting behaviors is helpful for the physician to determine what medication and what dosage would be appropriate.

## Inappropriate Sexual Behaviors

Conversations about sexual behaviors are avoided by many people, which is understandable. Inappropriate sexual behaviors are embarrassing to others while in public; you may avoid taking the person with dementia in public due to fear of embarrassment. If there is an inappropriate sexual behavior, check for a reason for the behavior without assuming it is a manifestation of dementia. For example, a person with dementia may take off clothing in public but may be doing so because the clothing is uncomfortable. The person with dementia lacks the judgment to be aware disrobing is occurring in public. Also, genitals may be exposed because the person needs to use the bathroom and is unable to communicate that need. I have heard of daughters caring for their father, who is sexually inappropriate because he recognizes her as his wife. Reorienting your loved one may be helpful, decrease embarrassment, and preserve dignity.

I mentioned a story earlier in the book of a minister who displayed hypersexual behaviors that were embarrassing to the family. Hypersexual behaviors occur more frequently in dementia that affect the frontal and temporal lobe. These behaviors can also come as the result of the need of human touch. Some people with dementia can be redirected by holding their hand and talking to them about a topic that distracts from the sexual behavior. I took care of a gentleman who was incredibly sweet but had frequent inappropriate sexual behaviors. He would pull my arm toward him and ask me to sit on his lap. I would tell him my husband would be upset with me if I did that. That comment seemed to ground him, and he would stop the behavior. Sometimes, ignoring the behavior is the best approach. I have a gentleman who can be very inappropriate when providing personal care, and I ignore the behavior all together. I continue to perform my job, but without acknowledging the behavior. He usually stops the behavior on his own. There are some people with dementia who masturbate, which can be troublesome for family. If this behavior occurs, it is best to allow the person you are caring for to be in a private area while performing this act. The same client I just mentioned started masturbating one evening I was caring for him. I walked away and gave him privacy. He did not remember masturbating, and I did not allow his behavior to affect my ability to care for him.

While touch and close connections with the person with dementia may decrease inappropriate sexual behaviors, it may not be enough for others. There is a class of medications known as selective serotonin reuptake inhibitors (SSRIs), which are used for depression but have the side effect of decreased libido. It may be worth trying if hypersexual behavior is affecting your loved one's daily life.

* * *

While some of these recommendations may work for you, some may not. There is not a one size fits all when it comes to caring for someone with dementia. For this reason, I encourage families of clients I care for to get involved with a dementia support group or take advantage of educational offerings from the Alzheimer's Association. This gives you the opportunity to meet other people who are having similar experiences. You can learn what they do to manage behaviors, and you may teach them something too.

# Chapter 5: Supported Self-Destruction

The disease might hide the person underneath
but there's still a person in there who needs
your love and attention.

—Jamie Calandriello

I received a call from the office stating that there was an inquiry call from a woman, Donna, who had many questions about services. Donna wanted to get services in place as soon as possible. I called Donna in between visits and could tell from that first call she was very anxious and uncertain of what was best for her mother. She indicated her eighty-three-year-old mother was losing weight and she was concerned about her overall health. Her mother had been living alone after losing her husband to Alzheimer's disease two years prior. Donna was also concerned because her mother indicated she did not feel capable of filling her medicine box and had asked the housekeeper to help. With Donna living in Massachusetts and her brother,

Jimmy, living in Colorado, helping their mother manage her medical needs was becoming increasingly difficult. Donna admittingly stated she believes that there are more health issues than she is aware of. I was also told her mother was very difficult and she is not sure her mother would accept the help. Several days after the call, I met Karen for the first time.

Karen was a petite woman with short, blonde hair. She dressed nicely but also comfortably. She was a little guarded but appeared appreciative of some help. Her voice was soft, and she smiled often. She lived in a modest home in a gated and guarded community. Soon after I arrived, she introduced her two cats. She told me how much she loves her cats and how much having them with her has been a help to her.

After doing a nursing assessment, I looked through all her medication and the box that was filled by her housekeeper. Although I am sure the housekeeper did her best, the medicine box was not filled appropriately. I filled her medicine box based on the most recent physician orders. When I asked questions about her past medical history, I could tell there were many gaps. There were also discrepancies between physician paperwork and instructions on medication bottles. She indicated she stopped a couple of medications, some at her judgment and others at the direction of her physician, which was documented. It was apparent a thorough medication reconciliation was needed.

Cognitive testing showed possible mild impairment versus early dementia. She reported she has been sleeping well, and with the many medication discrepancies, it was entirely possible her impairment was reversible. While reconciling her medications and ensuring all her physicians were receiving adequate information, I also reviewed medical records. Karen was seen by her PCP, Dr. Mercia, several times for diarrhea and was in the ER for continued diarrhea three months prior to our meeting. She was told to follow up with gastroenterology to investigate the cause further. She indicated she was not receiving calls to follow up and felt the medical system forgot about her. I did not know it at the time, but gastroenterology had been trying to follow up, but Karen was not able to manage her medical care.

I scheduled an appointment for a gastroenterologist, who ordered her to have sigmoidoscopy prior to the appointment since so much time had elapsed. Part of the preoperative process included a lab known as international normalized ratio (INR). Since she was on blood thinner, it was important to ensure her INR was normal before the procedure. Her INR came back high, which indicated her blood was too thin to have the procedure. When going through medications on my initial assessment, she indicated she was having her INR checked, and it had been stable for a long time. I had not anticipated this was going to be a barrier.

I took her home and she went straight to bed. She was hesitant to allow me to enter her room but knew she needed my help. Immediately after walking into her room, I noticed newspaper scattered on the carpet, from her bed to the bathroom. Without asking, she told me she was using newspaper to cover up areas where she had diarrhea. I walked into the bathroom and found even more newspaper. There was newspaper by her sinks, outside of the bathtub, and the entire space around her toilet. There were multiple layers of newspaper; with every episode of diarrhea, she put another newspaper down. She stated she was embarrassed and did not want me to see her floors. I told her I understood she is not feeling well and is doing the best she can. I was there to help her, no matter what that meant. I removed the newspaper in the bedroom and found multiple areas with dried feces. I cleaned her carpet the best I could and knew it would need a deep cleaning. The bottom layers of newspaper in the bathroom were stuck to the floor. I picked up as much as I could and then used soap, water, and a mop scrubber to get the rest of the newspaper up. It was heartbreaking to think of what she must have been experiencing over the past couple of months. She was exceptionally grateful for the cleaning, understanding, and my desire to help without judgment.

I contacted Dr. Mercia and was able to get Karen an appointment the next day. I contacted Donna to update her and commented about how gracious her mother was. Donna said in disbelief, "Really!" I was not provided with a lot of information when going in about two weeks prior and was mostly operating off what I saw and what I learned from Karen and her doctors.

Upon arriving the following day, Karen was ready to go but appeared very weak. She attempted to walk to the front door with her cane and nearly fell. Fortunately, I was next to her and was able to stabilize her. I told her we were not going to the doctor and that we needed to go to the ER. I felt like giving her an option may have led to the refusal for the ER because she had a concern for her cats whenever leaving the home. Arriving at the ER, I had to get a wheelchair for Karen. She was very weak and dizzy. While waiting for the doctor, we contacted her neighbor, who indicated she would care for Karen's cats while she was in the hospital. Karen was found to be in acute renal failure due to dehydration from diarrhea. Based on the labs, she would not have survived much longer under those conditions without emergency care. She was aggressively rehydrated while undergoing testing to determine the cause of diarrhea. She was found to have colitis, which can cause debilitating diarrhea but is treatable. In speaking with staff, I learned Karen had been given instructions each time she went to the clinic or upon discharge from the hospital but was not following up with orders. She had been blaming the system, but her cognitive impairment was preventing her from appropriate self-management. The staff was concerned about her cognition, as was her daughter, and it was decided Karen needed twenty-four-hour care, at least for the first week or two after hospitalization. After being in the hospital for four days, Karen was released home with twenty-four-hour care.

Around-the-clock care was very beneficial as Karen recovered and also allowed the care team to witness the extent of Karen's cognitive impairment and shifts in behaviors. Karen would insist all the lights in the house be turned off at night, which was respected, but challenging when staff needed to stay awake all night. Karen would periodically come out of her room in the middle of the night with a flashlight and go through the bedrooms. I do not know what she was looking for, but the staff indicated she seemed frantic. Karen checked the doors throughout the day and night to ensure they were locked. She stated that the doors need to remain locked so that the cats do not get out. She seemed to believe the cats could open doors if they were not locked.

As she felt better, the caregivers and I also witnessed a different personality emerge. Karen became angry and paranoid, which according to her daughter was the baseline personality. I finally understood the "Really!" comment when I indicated to Donna that her mother was gracious. Increased forgetfulness was noted, which intensified her anger. She stated she was not being kept up to date on changes and appointments. The truth was she did not remember that she did not remember. I attempted several methods of communication to help her feel in control to no avail. Any technology was refuted and too many reminders increased anger. She would call in the middle of the night, screaming that she did not know about an upcoming appointment and had no recollection of our previous conversations or my visits.

Karen became angry with me and yelled at one of my employees, stating that she should be ashamed to be working for a crook. A binder was kept in the home for caregiver communication and to keep information easily accessible. Since she associated the binder with me, she told my employee she was going to burn the binder. She attempted to burn the binder in her home. The caregiver was able to convince her to go outside if she needed to burn the binder.

Staffing was challenging because Karen would fire caregivers based on allegations that were nonsensical. One caregiver, who she adored, was told she is skating on thin ice because she "disconnected" the VCR. The caregiver stated she never touched the VCR, but Karen stated that was the only reasonable explanation. Some caregivers did not have the capacity to handle the erratic outbursts and did not want to work with Karen anymore. She also became angry about having someone in her home and convinced her children to decrease the care to six hours per day.

I received a call in the middle of the night to Karen screaming about her cats. She stated one of the caregivers was intentionally unlocking doors to help the cats escape. She also stated the same caregiver was coming to her home on nights she was not working and trying to open doors to let the cats out. Karen lived in a gated community, and when I asked about how the caregiver could do so, she stated the guards know the caregiver and just let her in. She stated that caregiver is not allowed back to her home. This was yet another caregiver that she adored and fired based on false information.

Karen's children were kept up-to-date on behaviors and attempts to help her feel in control and as independent as possible. Her son, Jimmy, suggested stopping her cholesterol medication, as it can cause cognitive impairment. After clearing that change with her physician, I performed cognitive testing, which indicated progression of altered cognition from the first assessment several months back. A cognitive test was repeated a month later to determine if there was a difference after the medication was stopped; there was no change.

Karen had a preventable hospitalization when she tried to manage her own care. I found out about her attempts after the fact. She again went home with twenty-four-hour care, with the same result in the end. Although there were many concerns about Karen's cognition, she continued to drive. The caregivers were not allowed to be a passenger in her vehicle, and since she insisted on driving, they would follow behind her in their vehicle. The caregivers were concerned about her driving and reported several instances that caused great concern. She was getting lost when driving in areas that were somewhat familiar in the past. She was late to many appointments as a result. Caregivers were frequently reporting that she was driving very close to other vehicles and that they were worried she would side swipe another car. There was an incident after leaving a restaurant when honking and yelling was heard by the caregiver. The caregiver stated a gentleman was directing his anger at Karen. She also saw a dent in the other car. Karen did not pay any attention to the gentleman and drove off. There were scratches on her car where she likely hit the other car.

## DRIVING WITH COGNITIVE IMPAIRMENT

I always recommend talking to your loved one about decisions that will need to be made as the disease progresses. This gives your loved one the ability to voice their desires and be a part of the decision-making process. When I am involved with this process, I ask my client how they will know it is no longer safe to drive. The response I generally get is, "I'll just know." I realize this is a difficult question. Driving is a part of our independence and losing that ability is an enormous loss. Is it time to give up driving when you get a ticket? Is it time when you forget where you are going? Is it time when you get into an accident? Most of my clients state that forgetting familiar areas when driving would be a concern. Too often than not this is not the reason a person with cognitive impairment stops driving. Keep reading: there will be a lot more information about driving considerations when cognitive impairment and dementia are present.

Dr. Mercia advised Karen to stop driving until a neurologist could further evaluate. This direction was not followed or enforced. In fact, her children stated she is safe to drive.

Jimmy came to town and had his mother drive him around. He concluded she was safe to drive and no further follow-up was necessary. I know her children were concerned about taking the vehicle away from their mother, and I can imagine they feared her anger all their life.

Karen was given a referral to see a neurologist, which initially was accepted by her. She stated if there is an issue, she wants to know about it and be treated. She later recanted after being told a report to the DMV could be filed if she is driving despite being told not to. Jimmy requested all neurology follow-up appointments be cancelled. Again, I believe this was due to his fear of his mother being angry with him. Meanwhile, there were continued episodes of confusion and paranoia. She started to have difficulty with her telephone. She would pick up the telephone, then when she heard the dial tone, she asked, "What is that?" She called another time in the middle of the night and the phone went to voicemail. I listened to the voicemail she left me. She was speaking nonsensically and seemed to be having a conversation with her cats. At the end of the call she said, "There, I did it," as if informing her cats of her followed instruction.

Several months later, Karen was back in the hospital. She was admitted once again, and the hospital staff had an opportunity to witness the extreme levels of confusion and paranoia that had been going on for months. While wearing her hospital gown and no socks, she left the building and was found in the parking lot looking for her car. It was winter at the time, and staff were concerned she did not have a safety awareness. She became very agitated and accusatory when security asked her to go back into the hospital building. She was eventually brought back to her room without incident. The staff was very concerned about her behavior, especially when coupled with consistent confusion.

Jimmy stated he wanted the neurology appointments back. It was too late, as they were cancelled when he requested previously. The wait time for neurology was several months, so we had to wait to start the process again. Prior to Karen being released from the hospital, the doctor ordered twenty-four-hour care. As history repeats itself, twenty-four-hour care did not last long. Jimmy backed the caregiving hours to eight hours per day. Jimmy also stated he wanted his mom to continue driving until there is a statement from a neurologist stating she cannot drive. Usually, a person does not drive until cleared, but Jimmy was advocating for the opposite.

A month later, Karen was back in the hospital for congestive heart failure. The hospital did a great job getting her back to her baseline, and she went back home with eight hours a day of care. We eventually got in with a neurologist who performed initial cognitive testing. The testing showed moderate to severe dementia. The neurologist stated my client should not drive until further testing can be done. I am sure you can guess what happened. She continued to drive and cancelled all neurological follow-up appointments. When I spoke to her children about the risk involved with her driving, they stated they were not concerned if she killed herself in an automobile accident. I asked them to think of the other drivers who could be seriously injured or killed with their mother behind the wheel. They stated they were willing to take that chance.

Karen's continued non-compliance and her children's lack of intervention put me in a dangerous position. At that point, it was my obligation to report Karen to the DMV. I also had to discontinue my services after providing ample notice and providing resources to Karen and Jimmy, who was already taking over the care management role. I can only hope Karen did not hurt herself or others in her driving crusade.

# Chapter 6:
# Where You Going with Those?

No love, no friendship can cross the path of our destiny without leaving some mark on it forever.

—François Mauriac

While I was starting my business, I contracted with an insurance company to case manage high-risk members. Most of the members had significant physical disabilities or an acute injury that made rehospitalizations probable. The goal of the program was to prevent unnecessary and preventable ER visits and manage health care in the community. If done correctly, the insurance company saves a great deal of money. When I was assigned members, I knew very little. I was responsible to set up my initial visit and complete a very thorough health history and determine needs.

Charles was pleased I would be coming over and helping him manage his health better. Charles lived in a community known as a continuing care retirement community (CCRC); he resided in the independent-living section. His apartment was small but sufficient for his needs. He had a kitchen, living room, bedroom, and one bathroom. Charles answered the door and politely asked me to enter, although I am not sure he remembered we had an appointment. He was about 6'2", thin framed, with tanned skin and white hair that appeared to have been cut using a bowl, literally. His bangs fell half-way between his scalp and eyebrows. He had a Southern drawl and was deliberate with his words.

## CONTINUING CARE RETIREMENT COMMUNITY

A CCRC, also known as a life plan community, are an all-in-one living option for seniors. The concept allows seniors to age in place in a different way. An aging adult can start in an independent setting, which could be a casita, villa, or apartment, depending on the facility. The independent setting has a large array of amenities, including dining, activities, and transportation. When the aging person needs more assistance, they can stay on the same campus of care but moved into an assisted living environment. At some point, an even higher level of care may be needed, at which time a skilled nursing facility (SNF) on campus is available. The SNF can also be a great place for short-term assistance after a hospitalization or surgery. Some communities also provide memory care, which is provided by healthcare professionals with specific dementia training.

Charles had been living in his apartment for about six months but still had boxes throughout the apartment as if he only unpacked half of his items. Charles was previously living with his wife; however, they were recently divorced. He and his wife were married for 54 years prior to getting a divorce.

I found it challenging to get through the assessment required by the insurance company. Charles often went on tangents and it took some skill to bring him back. I thought a cognitive issue may be present because he was repeating himself, but I did not want to assume this to be the case. I went back the next week to continue my initial assessment. I am not sure he remembered me, but he did graciously invite me inside. Our visits became more about his psychological needs and repetitive stories were expected. While addressing his emotional grief, I frequently redirected the conversation to address the health care aspects required by the insurance company.

Physically he was very healthy. He was able to perform his own activities of daily living (ADL), as well as his instrumental activities of daily living (IADL). Just because he was deemed independent with his IADLs, it does not mean he was doing so safely. He was on very few medications. He had mild chronic obstructive pulmonary disease (COPD), which was managed with an inhaler. He also had diet-controlled diabetes, high blood pressure, and high cholesterol. It was somewhat challenging to know what medications he was taking because he did not have a rational system in place, and I was concerned he was not taking medication as prescribed. The cognitive deficits were more apparent as my visits continued.

## ACTIVITIES OF DAILY LIVING & INSTRUMENTAL ACTIVITIES OF DAILY LIVING

ADLs and IADLs are aspects of functional status, which are evaluated when an individual appears to have a decline in their health. I prefer to use the Katz Index of Independence in Activities of Daily Living. There are six sections of functionality which include bathing, dressing, toileting, transferring, continence, and feeding. I also use the Lawton-Brody Instrumental Activities of Daily Living Scale. This scale has eight sections of functionality, which include ability to use a telephone, shopping, food preparation, housekeeping, laundry, mode of transportation, responsibility for own medications, and ability to handle finances. When caring for someone with dementia, I first notice difficulty with IADLs, and as the disease progresses, a person with dementia becomes completely dependent on others for IADLs. As complete dependence on IADLs is occurring, partial dependence on ADLs starts to occur. In the end stages of dementia, a person is completely dependent on others for all ADLs and IADLs.

Charles had a couple of stories that were imprinted in his brain. One involved his ex-wife. Charles stated he liked helping his neighbors, and when fruit would grow on his trees, he enjoyed picking the fruit and bringing it to his neighbors. He had a bicycle with a basket on the front to transport the fruit. Charles recalls walking through the living room with an arm full of fruit he had just picked from the backyard. He was transporting the fruit to his bicycle. His wife spotted him and asked, "Where you going with those?" which he described in a tone that was "real hateful like." His nose scrunched up when he made that statement. He concluded his wife disliked his desire to share their fruit with the neighbors. I heard this story on almost every visit.

Charles recalled another story, which involved his daughter. He stated they were having a regular conversation when, out of nowhere, his daughter said, "You said this and that was a lie. You also said this and that was a lie." He could not tell me what she thought he was lying about or tell me his response, but the story went the same way every time. I would attempt to talk to him about how these interactions were affecting him in his current life, but he did not seem to have the ability to elaborate outside of his scripted stories. The repetitive stories and difficulty with reasoning, concentration, and executive function were cause for concern.

Charles had difficulty managing his doctor's appointments, and it was clear he was not addressing his needs. Instead of my weekly visit to his apartment, I met him at his PCP appointment. As I walked toward the door, he was walking out. He stated that the office moved his appointment and that he is not going to be seen today. Since he drove himself there, he headed back to his apartment. I proceeded to the doctor's office to obtain more information. After confirming I had authorization to receive information, the receptionist indicated Charles comes to the office nearly every day, thinking he has an appointment. She stated they have been concerned about him and his ability to self-manage. I was able to find out when his next appointment was and put it on my schedule.

I made a visit to Charles the following week and wrote the upcoming appointment in multiple places throughout his apartment, hoping to keep him on track. During that visit, I noticed discharge paperwork from the hospital on his table. Initially, he did not remember going to the ER. I read through the paperwork and realized he had been to the ER since the last time I saw him. He then told me he had difficulty breathing and thought he was having complications from COPD, so he went to the hospital. It was noted in the ER Charles did not know how to use his inhaler when prompted to by the staff. No changes to his medication were made, and he was instructed to follow up with his physician. The reason he was on the program through the insurance company was to avoid visits to the ER. His cognitive impairment coupled with his infrequent doctor visits were to his detriment.

The morning of Charles's doctor's appointment, I called to remind him of the appointment and to let him I know was meeting him there. Apparently, the day prior, the office called to remind Charles of his appointment and he rescheduled. I showed up for his appointment and learned of the change; however, the visit was beneficial, as I was able to directly speak to his doctor. His doctor expressed deep concern about Charles's safety. He had been seeing Charles for over ten years and knew him quite well. It was as though he was pleading with me to do something to protect him. This is when I reached out to his daughter.

Charles's daughter, Janae, had a sweet voice and sounded genuinely concerned about her father. As I described what I was seeing, she validated this as being his normal behavior for the past two years. She stated her parents were living together until recently, but her mother had to ask him to leave because his cognitive impairment was disruptive, and he refused to seek assistance. Janae stated she has tried to help him, but getting him into independent living has been her only successful action. Janae knew her dad needed to be in assisted living, at a minimum, but she did not know where to turn. She also stated her dad thinks she is teaming up with her mother, his ex-wife. Janae did not know what he thought their plot was but knew he felt their intentions were malicious. Janae expressed emotional distress over the situation. I actively listened to her experience and elaborated on my involvement and concerns. We discussed the course of action she needed to take on his behalf to protect him. Fortunately, Janae had power of attorney and could make some steps.

Her first steps were to get involved with his medical appointments and to make sure he was completing the follow-up ordered by his physicians. I also encouraged her to get a neurologist for her dad. Charles still driving was another major concern. Driving is one of the most challenging aspects in dementia because it is difficult to know when a person with cognitive impairment should stop driving.

## DRIVING

Driving is a complex task that requires adequate peripheral vision, insight, and good judgement and the ability to make quick decisions. Driving is also an act of independence that is difficult for anyone to give up. A diagnosis of dementia does not mean that driving must cease, but it does mean that evaluation of safety must be done on an ongoing basis. A timely diagnosis allows for planning, which allows the person with dementia to be involved in decisions that will affect the future.

In a study to determine the risk of driving impairment caused by dementia, it was found persons with dementia were much more likely to fail a road test when compared to the healthy control. The study concluded even mild stages of dementia place people at a substantially higher risk of failing a performance-based road test and exhibit impaired driving abilities.

There are several warning signs to be cognizant about when determining if driving is safe. The most obvious warning sign is forgetfulness in familiar areas. Those with dementia tend to take the same route to familiar places, but when they cannot recall where to go, evidence shows the extent of damage to the brain may affect the ability to drive safely in general. Poor decision-making can be observed when the person with dementia is changing lanes without an awareness of other drivers, driving noticeably slower or faster than other drivers, failing to follow traffic signs and signals, parking inappropriately, driving into other lanes, and failure to signal in a suitable manner. There can also be confusion between the gas and brake pedal. Additionally, there may be irrational anger or increased nervousness or agitation when driving.

Conversations should begin early and involve family and close friends. Together, evaluation of safe driving and suitable options can be discussed. First and foremost, we must validate feelings associated with the loss of driving privileges. This is often the first major loss of independence that is followed by many other losses. Compassionate conversations should include desired transportation options, as well as practical steps to take as the disease progresses. Resistance in conversations about driving are common, as is resistance to enforcing actions that have been previously discussed. In some circumstances, a person with early-stage dementia may be willing to engage in conversations about how they would want intervention to occur when driving is deemed to no longer be a safe option. In most circumstances, this conversation is either highly opposed or not started early enough to have a positive impact.

With opposition, steps are needed to ensure the safety of the person with dementia. There may be opportunity to offer driving assistance. Many family members will provide transportation by simply stating they want to drive, communicating transportation is not a burden to them. There are transportation services for the elderly that can be prearranged. It is also advisable to consider a GPS for the vehicle to ensure you know where the vehicle is at any given time. While these are good first steps, it is likely the first step in a series of other steps to ensure safety.

With any change in the process, speak with the family physician and explain your concerns. The physician may be willing to write a prescription stating, "Do not drive." Just that alone may be enough. If driving continues, the physician may also request a medical driving assessment. A physician can also report an unsafe driver to the DMV. Check with the laws in your state about the specific assistance the DMV can provide. In some states a physician is required to file a report with the DMV if a diagnosis of dementia is given. If the physician is not comfortable with assisting, it may be necessary to seek out a geriatrician or neurologist.

Continued driving despite physician mandate puts the life of the person with dementia and others at physical risk but can also lead to litigation if an automobile accident takes place. If a person has been diagnosed with dementia and is in an accident, there is a significant risk to the driver with dementia. In the event of an accident, the automobile insurance is required to pay for any settlement or judgment up to the policy limits. With dementia, there is no additional coverage if the insurance company was not advised of the diagnosis. If a judgment is rendered over the amount of insurance liability, the insurance carrier would be responsible for any damages over the coverage limit. It is important to your loved one to understand the consequences of continued driving.

A more assertive approach is necessary if driving continues despite all other efforts to hinder driving. Car keys can be placed in possession of a trusted family member or friend or located in a concealed location. Disabling the car renders a vehicle unusable. This can be accomplished several ways, such as disconnecting the battery or removing leads from spark plugs. The vehicle itself may be a trigger; at which time, it should be removed from sight. The vehicle can be moved to a family member or friend's home or parked down the street if that is a safe option.

Some people choose to sell the car. If the person with dementia asks where the car is, a therapeutic fib, such as "The car is at the shop," can effectively impede any potential frustration. I have a client whose daughter disabled her car, which was necessary; however, she told her mother she did so and tried to explain why she made that decision. I highly discourage the honesty approach in this situation, as it will likely be one of the few memories the person with dementia remembers and will cause a strain on the relationship.

AARP (formerly known as the American Association of Retired Persons) has driving-assessment tools on their website. The Fitness-to-Drive Screening Measure Online was developed by the University of Florida, which assists in identifying at-risk drivers. There is also a program created in collaboration with the AARP, the American Automobile Association (AAA), and American Occupational Therapy Association (AOTA) called CarFit. There are events and virtual workshops to promote safe driving, to ensure the vehicle is the right fit, and to provide resources for driving safety.

As with any change occurring with dementia and the loss of independence, be supportive. Becoming more dependent on another person may bring about feelings of anger or sadness, and an empathetic approach validates the range of emotions that can be experienced. You may be asked questions about the vehicle or loss of driving multiple times, which can be frustrating. Framing your responses by contemplating how you would feel in the same situation will provide a compassionate approach.

Charles was more accepting of Janae's help than I thought he would be. Along with that also came arguments, as Charles wanted to continue living his life as he had, without the rationality or awareness of his own safety. Janae was able to move him to assisted living on the same campus he resided at. Assisted living provided twenty-four-hour supervision, medication management, transportation, and assistance with physician appointments. Janae continued meeting her dad at physician appointments and maintained communication between the medical providers and the facility. Charles was not pleased about the move initially, and while it was difficult for Janae to step in and make that decision for him, she knew she did what was in her dad's best interest. Janae was a fabulous advocate for her dad. As my business grew, I had to transition Charles to another case manager with the insurance company. I was grateful for the experience, and I'm confident Charles was in very good hands.

# Chapter 7:
# Resources to Provide Care

Of all the varieties of virtue, liberality is most beloved.

—Aristotle

There are government and private pay options to provide care wherever your loved one resides. Some of these services are used on an intermittent basis and others on a continuous basis. You will likely find, as the disease progresses, that you will utilize a variety of resources to enhance care and allow you time to care for yourself. I have met with many family members who are reluctant to use resources or would like to use resources but do not know where to turn. I have also worked with family members who want to do it all and do not seek resources until burnout occurs. You may find yourself reviewing this chapter multiple times as the disease progresses to ensure you are using all the resources available.

## MEDICARE

Medicare is a well-known national program, but most people know little about the benefit or have misconceptions about what Medicare can provide. Medicare has four parts, which include Medicare Part A, Medicare Part B, Medicare Part C, and Medicare Part D. Each will be discussed in detail in the following paragraphs. Medicare is available to those who are age sixty-five or older, people who are younger than sixty-five and have been receiving Social Security Disability benefits for twenty-four months (unless amyotrophic lateral sclerosis is present) or have permanent kidney failure requiring dialysis or a kidney transplant. For most people, initiation of Medicare benefits requires enrollment.

During the Initial Enrollment Period (IEP), a person who is within a seven-month period of their sixty-fifth birthday can sign up for Medicare Parts A and B. There is also a General Enrollment Period (GEP), which allows a beneficiary to sign up for Medicare if it was not completed during the IEP. The enrollment period for GEP is from January 1 to March 31. There is also a Special Enrollment Period (SEP), which is helpful for those who declined Medicare Part B because they or their spouse were still working and covered under an employer's health insurance plan. When enrolling in Medicare, a person is automatically provided Original, also known as traditional, Medicare. A person can choose at that time to receive benefits through a Medicare Advantage Plan. Beneficiaries can change the health plan during

Medicare Open Enrollment, which runs from October 15 to December 7 each year. Medicare cards display a social security number; however, this has been changed, and Medicare beneficiaries are now assigned a Medicare number.

## MEDICARE PART A

Medicare Part A benefits are available to beneficiaries for care at an inpatient hospital or post-hospitalization care, which includes skilled nursing facilities, home health care, and hospice services. Part A provides unlimited benefit periods that begin when the beneficiary is admitted to a hospital and ends when the beneficiary has not received acute or sub-acute care for sixty days. With that, if a beneficiary is hospitalized multiple times without a sixty day break between acute/sub-acute care, the benefit period continues. Medicare covers ninety days of inpatient care, in which a deductible is recovered by Medicare. Medicare also covers sixty lifetime reserve days, which are not renewable.

Hospice Part A covers room, board, care, and medical equipment if the facility participates in Medicare, a physician certifies that the beneficiary requires the level of care, the beneficiary has been hospitalized for at least three days in a row, and the beneficiary enters the facility within thirty days of discharge from the hospital. It is important to ensure hospital days are under an inpatient admission status. Hospital days in observation do not count toward the requirement. Check the Centers for Medicare & Medicaid Services website for deductible and coinsurance information, as these rates change annually.

Home health care, which encompasses skilled nursing and/or rehabilitation services, is covered under Medicare Part A if the beneficiary has a physician order indicating the need for specialized care in the home, the beneficiary receives at least one skilled service on an intermittent basis, the beneficiary is homebound, and the home care agency participates in Medicare. Skilled services include nursing, physical therapy, speech language pathology, and occupational therapy. Homebound status is a term indicating there is taxing effort to leave the home, but a person can leave the home for medical treatment, religious services, attend adult day care, or family gatherings, such as a funeral. Medicare does not have a limited number of visits if eligibility is met. Medicare does not collect a deductible or coinsurance for services under home health.

Hospice care is covered under Medicare Part A for beneficiaries who are certified by a physician to have a life expectancy of six months or less. Hospice provides a wide variety of services under the Medicare benefit; however, the beneficiary waives Medicare payments for outside services for the treatment of the terminal diagnosis. Hospice benefits include nursing care, medical social services, physician services, bereavement, chaplain services, short-term inpatient care, medications for palliative care, medical equipment, continuous home care, and respite care for caregivers. Short-term inpatient care and continuous care is only available if symptoms are not managed and a higher level of care is needed. Hospice contains two ninety-day certifications followed by unlimited sixty-day certifications. If the beneficiary continues to meet criteria, certifications continue, even beyond the six-month prognosis. Hospice services can be revoked and restarted later or can be discontinued by the hospice if criteria are no longer met for recertification.

## MEDICARE PART B

Medicare Part B covers a variety of necessary medical services, medical supplies that are not covered by other insurance, and medical equipment. Part B typically covers 80 percent for Medicare-approved services and beneficiaries are responsible for 20 percent. Some of the services covered under Part B include physician visits, outpatient services, laboratory services, and some medications. Under Medicare Part B, most prevention and screening services are covered, and the beneficiary does not have a financial obligation. Examples of these services include an annual wellness exam, bone mass screening, mammography, colorectal screening, prostate cancer screening, cervical and vaginal cancer screening, and the flu and pneumococcal immunizations. Services such as routine eye or hearing exams, hearing aids, most medications, private duty in-home care, and dental care are generally not covered under Medicare Part B.

Some beneficiaries choose additional coverage or a Medicare Advantage Plan to have coverage of services not covered by Medicare Part B. Check the Centers for Medicare & Medicaid Services website for *Medicare & You*. Some providers do not accept Medicare and can charge up to 15 percent more than the Medicare approved amount. I have seen more psychiatrists move away from Medicare and are either private pay only or take payment up front and submit the claim to insurance for a reimbursement to the beneficiary. Although durable medical equipment is covered, the process can be lengthy, and many people choose to purchase some equipment out of pocket as it is needed immediately. You should also be aware that Medicare may deny a claim for ambulance services. Medicare stipulates ambulance services must be used under certain circumstances, so if another mode of transportation would not have resulted in harm, the use of ambulance services was not warranted.

Additional Medicare coverage is available by several methods. Some retired individuals are provided with supplemental coverage; however, the percentage of people who have this benefit is decreasing as many companies are not offering retiree health coverage. Some beneficiaries acquire a Medicare supplement policy, also known as Medigap, which is obtained through a private insurance company. These policies are intended to fill the gaps of traditional Medicare, such as deductibles, coinsurance, excess charges, and some uncovered services. Medigap policies are identified by letters A, B, C, D, F, G, K, L, M, and N, depending on the state you live in. As with any insurance, the less expensive the policy the smaller the coverage. Claims are first sent to Medicare and then the excess is sent to the supplemental insurance. If Medicare does not cover a claim, the supplemental insurance does not cover the claim. Military retires, their family members and survivors, and some former spouses are eligible for TRICARE for Life. These policies cover much of what Medicare does not. I have cared for many clients who have Medicare and TRICARE for Life and can say this combination is the best insurance one can get and is well deserved. Lastly, some individuals receive Medicare and Medicaid services at the same time. Medicaid aids individuals who meet income and asset requirements. This is intended to assist those who otherwise would not be able to afford health-care services under traditional Medicare.

## MEDICARE PART C

Medicare Part C, also known as the Medicare Advantage program, enables beneficiaries to receive Medicare benefits through a private health plan. Medicare Advantage Plans provide the benefits available under traditional Medicare, except hospice; however, it has differences, such as prior approval and preauthorization procedures. One of the benefits of a Medicare Advantage Plan is the inclusion of benefits not covered under traditional Medicare, such as dental and vision care. Some plans also include prescription drug coverage. In terms of care for a person with dementia, benefits under a Medicare Advantage Plan can also include adult day care, home modifications, personal emergency response systems, respite care, personal home care, homemaker services, and meal delivery.

The main types of private health plans for Medicare Advantage include health maintenance organization (HMO), HMO with Point-of-Service (POS) option, preferred provider organization (PPO), Private Fee-For-Service (PFFS) plan, Special Needs Plan (SNP), and Medical Savings Account (MSA) plans. Enrollment in a Medicare Advantage plan occurs during open enrollment, from October 15 to December 7. Beneficiaries can switch from traditional Medicare to a Medicare Advantage plan, switch back to traditional Medicare from an Advantage plan, or switch Medicare Advantage plans. Beneficiaries also have a six-week period from January 1 to February 14 to switch from a Medicare Advantage plan to traditional Medicare, as well as enroll in Medicare Part D. There are provisions for changes during exceptional circumstances.

The Centers for Medicare & Medicaid Services rates Medicare Advantage programs with a star rating, which can be viewed on their website. In my experience, these plans work well if care is not required in the home. For example, after discharge from a hospital, the benefit would be very limited for physical therapy through home health, but coverage at an outpatient physical therapy center would be advantageous. For those who are homebound or anticipate a homebound status soon, a Medicare Advantage plan may be too restrictive and not provide the level of care that would be needed if you cannot leave the home for health care.

## MEDICARE PART D

Medicare Part D is provided through private insurance companies to provide prescription drug plans. There are also phases to Medicare Part D coverage. The first phase is the deductible period, where the beneficiary pays 100 percent of medication costs until the deductible is met. The beneficiary then enters the initial coverage period, in which the plan will pay for a portion of medications and the beneficiary pays a copayment. Once the beneficiary has accumulated a specific dollar amount in total medication costs, the beneficiary enters the coverage gap, which is also known as the donut hole. In the donut hole the beneficiary would be required to pay a larger portion of the prescription drug costs until the beneficiary reaches the yearly out-of-pocket spending limit. This changed in 2020: the donut hole closed for all prescription drugs. In the coverage gap, the beneficiary is responsible for 25 percent of the cost of drugs. The last phase is the catastrophic coverage, where the beneficiary pays significantly lower copayments for medications once a spending threshold has been met.

There are also four tiers for medication coverage, with generic medications usually being the lowest co-payments and non-formulary medication more costly. Since the deductible amounts change, you will want to check your plan for specific information. The Extra Help program provides financial assistance to beneficiaries with low income to assist in paying for Part D plan premiums and cost-sharing charges. People who have benefits through Medicare and Medicaid or Supplemental Security Income (SSI) are automatically enrolled in the Extra Help program.

When Medicare denies payment for a service, Medicare beneficiaries have the right to file an appeal. When a provider anticipates a specific service may not be covered under Medicare, you should be issued an Advance Beneficiary Notice (ABN) or Notice of Medicare Noncoverage (NOMNC). A provider cannot bill for a service associated with a denied claim if the beneficiary did not agree to the service under an ABN or NOMNC. Additionally, when a Medicare beneficiary is being discharged from a facility billing under Medicare, the beneficiary has the right to appeal the decision for discharge. This occurs most frequently when a person is hospitalized and does not feel the discharge decision is appropriate and continued hospital care is needed. Be advised: if the decision is upheld by Medicare, you may be responsible for the costs associated with extending care in the hospital or facility.

## MISCONCEPTIONS ABOUT MEDICARE

There are a few misconceptions about Medicare you should be aware of. The first is that Medicare will cover long-term care. While Medicare does cover short-term admissions in a skilled environment, Medicare does not cover indefinite care in a facility. For example, if a person is in a rehabilitation center under Medicare and has reached rehab potential, Medicare will no longer cover the costs of this level of care. While some people choose to remain in the long-term care setting for a variety of reasons, doing so would not be covered under Medicare. Medicare does not cover non-skilled or custodial care. I have spoken with many people on the phone that read the benefits guide from Medicare that include a section indicating Medicare will pay for twenty-four-hour care. This is misleading, not purposefully, as Medicare does pay for twenty-four-hour care in a facility under certain circumstances, but again, this is on a short-term basis.

Another misconception is Medicare has been adversely affected by the Affordable Care Act (ACA). ACA expanded preventative services and changed the coverage gap in Part D to the advantage of the beneficiary. I have also heard clients comment they will ask their doctor about Medicare coverage. Although doctors are very knowledgeable, their ability to help guide you through Medicare decisions is very limited. Lastly, some people believe Medicare Part D will pay for all prescriptions. Some medications are excluded from coverage, as well as most over the counter medications. Medicare Part D pays a portion of drug costs.

## MEDICAID

Medicaid is a national health-insurance program for people with low income, which operates as a federal-state partnership. Since Medicaid is a needs-based program, applicants must prove financial necessity by demonstrating assets and income are low enough to meet the program's eligibility standards, which varies by state. Each state administers their own Medicaid program under broad federal rules with oversight from the Centers for Medicare & Medicaid Services.

As mentioned previously, Medicare beneficiaries can be dual-eligible for Medicaid services. All state Medicaid programs offer a Medicare Savings Program, which helps pay Medicare premiums for those with low income who meet qualifications for the program. Mandatory services under Medicaid include physician services, hospital services, nursing facility services, home health care, transportation services, laboratory, and imaging services. Some Medicaid programs also cover long-term care, custodial care, dental services, rehabilitation, case management, respiratory care for ventilator-dependent individuals, hospice, private-duty nursing, prosthetic devices, eyeglasses, and durable medical equipment.

Medicaid does not have a specific enrollment period. There is a process to evaluate financial resources, such as income and assets, while also considering excluded financial resources. There may also be a process to determine eligibility based on medical necessity, for those who are dual-eligible. Some people spend down financial resources to qualify for the program, which is a legally acceptable method to use countable resources to purchase exempt resources. An older adult applying for Medicaid must be able to prove assets were not transferred during a sixty-month look-back period. An elder law attorney can prove helpful in retaining assets for needed care, while also qualifying for state assistance.

There are also non-Medicaid assistance programs that are state-funded or state-managed, which are designed for low-income individuals that require assistance with activities of daily living. Some states have additional generalized assistance programs that are designed specifically for individuals with dementia.

## SOCIAL SECURITY

Social Security is a well-known benefit for those who are retired and who are at least sixty-two years of age. Benefits are available based on wages or self-employment income in a calendar year. Social Security also offers survivor benefits, which provide 75–100 percent of the deceased's basic Social Security benefit to a widower, qualified divorced spouse, children, and dependent parents. The survivor benefit is meant to supplement support that was provided by the deceased's income. Even though the minimum age to begin collecting Social Security is sixty-two, many individuals wait until ages sixty-five to sixty-seven to receive a higher benefit payment. Some individuals choose to increase the amount of their monthly benefit by delaying retirement until the age of seventy. At age seventy, the maximum benefit would be received. Some individuals choose to continue working while drawing Social Security benefits as well. Some people do have to pay federal income taxes from the Social Security benefit.

Social Security Disability Insurance provides partial replacement of income before retirement to those who cannot participate in substantial employment as the result of a severe disability, which can be physical or mental. This benefit may be especially important for those diagnosed with an early-onset dementia that affects the person to the extent employment is no longer feasible. The individual must meet eligibility requirements, such as gainful employment contributing to Social Security for at least five of the last ten years before the disability. Beneficiaries who receive Social Security Disability benefits for twenty-four months are eligible for benefits under Medicare, regardless of their age.

SSI is a federal program that provides a monthly income for those with low income and limited financial resources. The benefit is determined based on a percentage of the federal poverty level. Some states also supplement the federal SSI benefit. In most states, SSI beneficiaries are also eligible for their state's Supplemental Nutrition Assistance Program (SNAP).

Applicants can apply for benefits with the Social Security Administration by calling or completing an online application. Applicants can also visit their local Social Security office after setting up an appointment.

## Veteran Benefits

Many veterans or surviving spouses are not aware of the various benefits available through Veteran Affairs (VA). Benefit programs have two eligibility requirements: a qualifying service record and at least one day of wartime service. A qualifying service record entails discharge from active-duty service under conditions other than dishonorable. Wartime periods include WWII (December 7, 1941–December 31, 1946), Korean War (June 27, 1950–January 31, 1955), Vietnam War (February 28, 1961–May 7, 1975, for veterans who served in the Republic of Vietnam; and August 5, 1964–May 7, 1975, for veterans who served outside the Republic of Vietnam), and Gulf War (August 2, 1990 through a date to be set by law or presidential proclamation). Some VA benefits also require the veteran to be age sixty-five or older.

The VA pension benefit provides tax-free supplemental income to wartime veterans or their families with insufficient income to meet their basic needs. There are three pension levels. Level 1 is a basic pension. The veteran requirement is at least ninety days of active-duty service, discharge other than dishonorable conditions, income test (adjusted yearly net income is below the maximum annual pension rate), financial net worth (assets do not exceed the countable net worth limitations), and age or disability criteria. Age or disability criteria must be met by an age of sixty-five or older, a permanent and total nonservice-connected disability, or receiving SSDI/SSI benefits. Level 2 is housebound or midlevel pension. The veteran qualifications include all requirements for the basic pension and VA housebound criteria, which means the veteran or surviving dependent must be significantly confined in the home environment due to a permanent disability. Level 3 is aid and attendance pension and is the highest level of pension benefits. The veteran or surviving dependent must meet basic pension requirements and depend on others for care. Dependance on others for care is determined by the need for assistance with activities of daily living (bathing, dressing, mobility, toileting, and continence) and if the person is bedridden, living in a skilled environment due to a mental or physical incapacity, or is blind.

The VA works with the IRS and Social Security to verify beneficiaries continued eligibility from a financial standpoint. With frequent changes to financial aspects of eligibility, it is best to refer to the U.S. Department of Veteran Affairs website.

Another underutilized veteran benefit is Service-Connected Disability Compensation. A common misconception of the benefit is for soldiers wounded in action, but the benefit is much broader. The VA recognizes many disabilities and diseases, which are expanded regularly. It is more common nowadays for a veteran to apply to disability compensation immediately following the date of separation from service. Those who served many years ago may not be aware of their eligibility to receive compensation benefits. To qualify, the veteran must prove their disability or disease was the consequence of or aggravated by military service. This is completed by reviewing medical records and through a medical examination. The VA uses a scale of 0–100 percent, which corresponds to the severity of the disability. Rating percentages adjust in 10 percent increments. If a condition has worsened, a veteran may request the VA to redetermine disability to potentially obtain a higher disability rating. This should be done with caution as the VA may not agree the condition has worsened and may also determine other conditions under compensation have improved, which could decrease the disability rating.

There are presumptive conditions in which a veteran who is diagnosed with a disability or disease and served in a location where the environment may have caused the disability or disease, so VA disability compensation is awarded. For example, my father was hospitalized several times for an embolus (blood clot) in his legs. Upon running tests, my father was told he had leukemia. Further testing showed he was diagnosed with hairy cell leukemia. Presumptively, hairy cell leukemia is caused by Agent Orange, which was used during the Vietnam War. My father was a veteran of the Vietnam War, and as such, he received VA disability compensation. The VA also provided medical care for the condition at no cost to him. Fortunately, it was caught early, and he got through treatment beautifully.

The VA operates the nation's largest integrated health-care system. Some veterans use the VA health-care system exclusively, some use Medicare or health insurance in addition to VA health-care benefits, while some veterans do not use the VA health-care system at all. To qualify, a veteran must have served active-duty military and been discharged for other than dishonorable reasons. A veteran is required to submit VA Form 10-10EQ and will then begin the enrollment process. The level of health-care services under the VA is determined by veteran's disabilities (disability rating), income, and net worth. The VA operates hospitals, health clinics, and pharmacies across the country. Based on the priority level, some veterans are also provided with dental and vision benefits as well. It is recommended that a veteran does enroll in the VA health-care system, if eligible, even if another health insurance will be utilized and health care will be obtained outside of the VA system, as long-term benefits require a veteran to be enrolled in the health-care system. It is best to do so before the need arises, as processes within the VA system can be time-consuming.

As mentioned, TRICARE for Life (TFL) is a health-insurance and care program for retired members and family of all seven uniformed services. TFL picks up where Medicare leaves off. There is also the Civilian Health and Medical Program of the Department of Veterans Affairs (CHAMPVA), which is intended for spouses and/or children of veterans permanently disabled or killed in the line of duty. This program is beneficial for those who are not eligible for TRICARE.

Veterans enrolled in the VA health-care system are eligible for home- and community-based service benefits if there is a medical need for the assistance. A VA physician will determine if there is a need and can then order the necessary services. Services include respite care (thirty days per year for caregivers), VA nursing homes (first reserved for veterans with a service-connected disability), hospice and palliative care, medical foster homes, assisted living, geriatric evaluation, adult day health programs, skilled home health care, and Program of All-Inclusive Care for the Elderly (PACE).

Veterans may receive Medicaid services while receiving VA benefits. The balance between the benefits can be tricky. There are situations in which applying for one benefit program can lead to an imposed penalty or denial of benefits from another program. I recommend consulting with an attorney with VA benefit experience or a VA accredited professional. A professional can ensure you are using the right benefits to maximize long-term benefits.

Eligible veterans and dependents can request to be buried at a national cemetery operated by the VA. The benefit covers the cost of the gravesite and the opening and closing of the grave. A veteran may also be eligible to receive a government headstone or marker, a burial flag, and a presidential memorial certificate regardless of the place of burial. These benefits are provided at no cost to the veteran's family. If the veteran qualifies for the VA burial and memorial benefits, the veteran's spouse and dependent children may also be buried in a VA national cemetery.

## DEPENDENT-CARE ACCOUNTS

A dependent-care account is a type of flexible spending account (FSA) that is part of an employer benefit plan. This type of FSA is generally used for childcare, but it can also be used for in-home caregivers or a senior or adult day care. An employee can put aside a limited amount in pre-tax dollars into a dependent-care account to assist with dependent-care expenses. The limited amount that can be put into an FSA changes, so it is best to ask your employer what the current limit is. If you can get an FSA through your employer, it is important to remember the money must be spent in the calendar year, because it does not roll over.

## TAX DEDUCTIONS

The Tax Credit for the Elderly and Disabled is a tax credit for persons over age sixty-five or for persons under sixty-five who are disabled. The credit has eligibility limits based on adjusted gross income. The credit is applied to a tax filer's return, so an aging parent who is claimed as a dependent on someone else's tax return is not eligible. In some situations, it may be beneficial to forego the Elderly and Disabled Tax Credit and have the elderly or disabled individual claimed as a dependent on the tax return.

The Child and Dependent Care Credit is also known as the Elderly Dependent Care Credit or Aging Parent Tax Credit. It is a tax credit for expenses a person or family incurs while caring for a dependent to allow the taxpayer the freedom to work. The paid services applied to the Dependent Care Credit cannot also be used for a medical expense deduction. It is advisable to use a tax preparation service to maximize the Dependent Care Credit. Some states also offer tax credits for dependent care.

Medical expenses can be deducted if the total sum exceeds a percentage of the tax filer's adjusted gross income, if sixty-five years or older, or exceed a higher percentage of the adjusted gross income for those sixty-four or younger. To claim an individual under your care, the tax filer must provide more than half of the dependent's financial support and the dependent must be related to or have lived with the tax filer for a full calendar year. Eligible medical and dental expenses include, but are not limited to, medical fees, cost of transportation for medical care, health insurance premiums, long-term care insurance, home modifications, personal care items, prescription medications, facility entrance fees, and room and board for assisted living if assistance with activities of daily living are needed. Consult with a tax professional to determine the current percentage of the tax filer's adjusted gross income used in the calculation.

## Reverse Mortgage

A reverse mortgage is a cash loan that is taken against the home equity. The lending bank makes payments in a single lump sum, in monthly installments, or as a line of credit. The loan is not paid back until the home is sold, the last borrower passes away or moves from the home after one year. Usually, the loan is not paid back and when the home is sold, the lender is paid back the loan amount plus interest. The reverse mortgage relevant to the elderly is the Home Equity Conversion Mortgage (HECM). The loan is insured by the United States federal government and is only accessible by a lender who is approved by the Federal Housing Administration (FHA).

When a senior is in a situation where they do not have the income or savings to pay for care, home modifications, or long-term care insurance, a reverse mortgage can provide financial resources to continue to age in place. At times, the funds are used to purchase long-term care insurance; however, the best time to purchase long-term care insurance is long before assistance is needed or anticipated. The longer you wait to get long-term care insurance, the more costly the policy will be. It is not uncommon for funds from a reverse mortgage to be used for a family member to provide care in the home. This is feasible when a family member is providing care and, as a result, is not able to maintain employment.

Commonly used government benefits are not affected by a reverse mortgage, such as Medicare and Social Security. Some programs, such as SSI, Medicaid, and Veterans Pension eligibility may be affected. The impact of a reverse mortgage on government benefits varies by state. Payments from a reverse mortgage are not counted as income if they are spent in the same month as they are received.

Requirements for a reverse mortgage include an age of sixty-two or older, financial capability to maintain the home, paying taxes and insurance, and a history of paying bills timely. There are no requirements for health status, marital status, and geographic location. The home must be the senior's primary residence. The reverse mortgage must be the primary debt against the house. Homes of any value can qualify; however, there are limits on how much can be borrowed. The property must be a single-family home, a two-to-four-unit home with one unit occupied by the borrower, a HUD-approved condominium, or an FHA approved manufactured home. It is important to remember, a reverse mortgage salesperson is not a financial planner or expected to know eldercare needs and may not have your best interest in mind. It would be wise to speak with an approved reverse mortgage counselor or your financial advisor.

The HUD exchange can provide phone or face-to-face meetings with a counselor to fully understand the benefits and limitations of a reverse mortgage. There are financial alternatives to a reverse mortgage, such as a line of credit, which may be a more suitable option, depending on the overall financial picture.

## Long-Term Care Insurance

Long-Term Care Insurance is a policy that pays for some or all senior long-term care costs. These policies require a monthly premium and can be used for services at home, in adult day care, and in assisted living or in skilled facilities. Typically, these policies are taken out prior to the age of sixty and prior to debilitating illness requiring assistance. Long-Term Care Insurance is not intended for someone who has immediate health needs requiring assistance. Long-Term Care Insurance plans vary greatly. For the purposes of this book, I will discuss what you need to know if your loved one has a policy that you will need to use now or at some point in the disease process. If your loved one has dementia, this would not be the time to purchase a policy.

When I work with families, one of the first questions I ask is if there is a Long-Term Care Insurance policy. Many family members are not sure if their loved one has a policy. If time permits, it is important to ask about a Long-Term Care Insurance policy prior to disease progression. If you have taken over bill payment, you may notice a recurring payment to an insurance company or you may be receiving bills.

When calling a Long-Term Care Insurance company, there are some important questions you will need to ask to understand the benefit. You should first inquire what the process is to open a claim. Some companies send an assessor to the home to determine if the insured does require assistance for a disability or disease. For some, the assessment is completed over the phone. You will want to determine if the policy has an elimination period, which requires the insured to privately pay for care prior to the policy being used. If there is an elimination period, you will want to know if there is a certain number of days and/or hours care must be received prior to the policy paying for care. Each plan has a care allowance, which can vary greatly. Some policies have a daily maximum, and some have a monthly maximum. The care allowance may be different depending on what type of care is being provided and the location of care services. You should also inquire about the length of the payout duration. Some policies cover benefits for a certain number of years, while others are unlimited. The payout duration may also depend on the level of care, such as at home or in a facility. Some policies also cover intermittent home nursing services and equipment needed to provide care, such as a wheelchair. Some of the newer policies also have a life insurance benefit, where money not spent on care can be dispersed to a beneficiary upon death.

## LIFE INSURANCE

If your loved one has a life insurance policy but need money to pay for care, a life settlement may be a good option. The purchaser of the policy pays future premiums and collects the death benefit upon maturity—that is, the purchaser becomes the beneficiary of the policy. Some factors that increase the life settlement payout include advanced age of the insured, short life expectancy (not necessarily terminally ill), lower cash surrender value as a percent of the coverage amount, and lower annual premiums as a percent of the coverage amount. The qualifications for life settlements vary greatly; a life settlement broker can assist in selling the policy for a fee.

With a life insurance policy, there is also the option to obtain a death benefit loan, which is taken against the cash value of the policy, not against the death benefit amount. These loans have a low interest rate and do not have repayment schedules. An accelerated death benefit allows a life-insurance-policy owner to receive a portion of their death benefit from the insurance company. Generally, the policyholder must be terminally ill. The benefit does not need to be repaid. The loan amount is deducted from the face value when the death benefit becomes due.

A viatical settlement is another option to obtain a lump sum of cash for a life insurance policy. The difference with a viatical settlement is that life expectancy is much longer. This can be helpful when a person is trying to qualify for Medicaid, as an insurance policy with a death benefit greater than $1,500 is considered a countable asset. This asset can cause a person to be denied Medicaid benefits. A viatical settlement could also change the financial status of the individual and affect SSI, Medicaid, and other assistance programs. The benefits and consequences should be weighed to determine if a viatical settlement is a feasible option.

A Life Insurance Conversion allows the sale of a life insurance to a third party to receive money for long-term care services or home modifications. This program is specifically structured to allow policy holders to gain Medicaid eligibility. The buyer of the policy takes over the monthly premiums, pays the care providers' fees, and collects the death benefit when the policyholder passes.

## COMMUNITY SUPPORT

The Alzheimer's Foundation of America provides respite grants to non-profit member organizations, who in turn work directly with families to administer the grants. The

Alzheimer's Association also has a Respite Grant Program, which is administered by the local chapters. You should check with the local agency to determine eligibility and availability. The care recipient must have a diagnosis of Alzheimer's disease or related dementia. There may also be age, financial, geographic, and caregiver-specific requirements to qualify. These programs are intended to provide resources for respite care but do not address long-term care needs.

* * *

The resources discussed are not intended to specifically guide you on the best benefits for your loved one. It is an overview of resources for you to consider. Speak with a specialist to determine the most feasible intervention for your situation.

# CHAPTER 8:
## TILL DEATH DO US PART

We remember their LOVE
when they can no longer remember.

—Anonymous

William and Donna had been married for nearly thirty years. The Petersons hid a precarious life behind the closed doors of the home they owned since they were married. Their health was deteriorating from various ailments, each with strengths that helped the other stay in their home. They were oblivious to their son's intrusion inside of their home. Their adult son, who was a known drug abuser and frequently incarcerated, had been living with them. He occupied an 11 x 12 foot space and they rarely saw him. The Petersons' neighbors, who were close friends for many years, were growing increasingly concerned about their health and had a gut feeling something was wrong. They contacted Adult Protective Services (APS) to allow an evaluation to determine if the Petersons' were in a predicament they could not see or avoid.

APS visited the home and conducted an evaluation. Not only were there concerns about the Petersons' health and ability to care for themselves, but there was also evidence their son, Nathan, was abusing the Petersons. Upon further investigation, it was discovered Nathan was stealing large sums of money from his parents, likely to purchase illicit drugs. The investigator also discovered the presence of fourteen dogs, two birds (in cages), and seven caged gerbils. The 11 x 12 room was full of garbage and feces and smelled like urine. The presence of this occurring in their home without any knowledge made the Petersons' situation even more suspicious.

The only other family the Petersons had was a niece, Megan, who lived locally but had a busy career and a family; Megan had not been that involved with her aunt and uncle. With the extent of cognitive impairment and lack of power of attorney, Megan was asked to assist. As mentioned previously, in the absence of a power of attorney and the Petersons' inability to appoint one due to cognitive impairment, the court was petitioned to appoint a guardian and conservator. Since Megan was willing and able, she was eventually appointed and was named the legal representative. One of the first actions was evicting Nathan from the home. Once it was safe for my involvement, Megan asked me to assist William with management of his care, while keeping an eye on Donna to ensure she was safe.

Megan met me at the Petersons' home to introduce me and explain my role in their care. Donna answered the door and graciously allowed us to enter. She was wearing a pinstripe pant suit, black heels, and bold jewelry. Her hair was teased like she just walked out of the 1980s, and she was wearing very colorful makeup. She appeared to have worked hard to prepare for the initial meeting. William was already in the living room, waiting for us to join him. He was obviously much older than Donna. Donna was in her early sixties and William twenty-five years her senior. William had a full head of gray hair that had a nice wave to it. He was wearing very short corduroy shorts with a polo shirt and shoes without socks. He appeared to enjoy tanning, as his skin was dark and leathery.

I was told Donna was an active alcoholic and suffered from cognitive impairment secondary to chronic alcohol abuse. Even though she presented well initially, her cognitive impairment was obvious once she spoke. She had a severe stuttering impediment, and her conversations were repetitive. She also used bizarre phrases, which I later coined as "Donna-isms." Donna was annoyed by my role, as she felt she was caring for her husband adequately. I do believe she did her best to care for William.

At eighty-seven, William had health issues common with older age; however, the most debilitating of his ailments was a CVA (stroke), which occurred two years prior to my involvement. Apparently, emergency services were refused by William after the stroke. Donna stated she wanted to call 911 but honored her husband's wish to be left alone. It was two days before a neighbor came over and called 911.

When a stroke occurs, time is of the essence. When an ischemic stroke occurs, emergency services are needed within six hours for optimal results. Because of the lapse, deficits remained until the day he died. He walked with a walker; he would push the walker about three feet away from him, leaving him with a slouched position when he ambulated. The deficits of the stroke caused left-sided weakness, so his left foot would drag behind him. It was a challenge for him to walk, and he was having many falls. He also suffered from vascular dementia because of the stroke.

### CEREBRAL VASCULAR ACCIDENT (CVA)

A stroke can be categorized as ischemic or hemorrhagic. Ischemic strokes are more common and are the result of a lack of blood flow to a region of the brain. A hemorrhagic stroke occurs when blood from an artery bleeds into the brain. Symptoms of either stroke depend on the area of the brain affected. Additionally, one side of the brain controls the opposite side of the body, so a stroke affecting one side of the brain will result in neurological complications on the other side of the body. If the affected area is the left brain, the right side of the body will be affected. This can be seen with paralysis or weakness on the right side of the body, speech and language difficulties, cautious behaviors, and memory loss. If the affected area is to the right side of the brain, the left side of the body will be affected. This can be seen with paralysis to the left side of the body, vision problems, impulsive behaviors, and memory loss. In some cases, a stroke occurs in the brain stem, which can leave the victim in a frozen-like state, where there is no speech or movement below the neck.

I began to manage William's medications as there was suspicion of inappropriate medication management. The first time I filled his medicine box I could tell he was not following physician orders. I had the bottles in front of me and noticed one of his blood pressure medication bottles had more than it should. I counted the pills remaining in the bottle and compared it to the amount dispensed. Based on my count, William missed half of his doses of one of his blood pressure medications. He told me he did not need help with his medication because he could do it himself. He said he did not miss one dose. I responded, "You're right. You missed fifteen doses." I was able to show him my findings and then he was a little more accepting. In the beginning, I was filling his medication boxes and leaving the bottles in the home. I came to realize that either he or Donna were getting into the bottles and moving medications around. With permission from his niece, I took the medication bottles out of the home. I would fill a medication box prior to arriving and switch it out with an empty box. We continued this cycle, although he and his wife were not happy. Donna would call the office stating she needs the bottles to be brought back immediately. I realize this was due to her lack of control and loss of independence.

William was a cantankerous man who was angry about his circumstances and inability to change the course. His difficulty hearing made communication even more difficult. William was annoyed by his wife's mere presence. I recall being in the living room when she brought him a sandwich for lunch; he took one bite, spit it out, and commented on how horrible it tasted. He told her to go back to the kitchen and make something else. Donna was a self-proclaimed chef; however, William complained about every bit of food she brought him. William was also irritated by the five dogs living in the home. He did whatever he could to stay away from the dogs.

At some point I became concerned about William and Donna's vulnerability to scams. They were receiving multiple calls from people they did not know, and I was seeing mail on their table that seemed deceiving. One day, as I checked their mail, I noticed a letter William put in the mailbox to be picked up by the postal carrier, in which he placed cash to be entered into a drawing. Elderly people in general are vulnerable to scams. The presence of cognitive impairment increases the vulnerability.

## SENIOR SCAMS

Senior scams are an increasingly problematic issue and knowing what to look out for and how to respond is critical. According to the FBI, seniors are likely targets for several reasons. One of the most obvious is the higher probability an older person is to have altered cognition and problems with short-term memory. Seniors may also be reluctant to report possible scams out of fear of being viewed as lacking mental capacity. A senior may also feel ashamed they fell for a scam. Lastly, many seniors develop a "nest egg" and thrive on building excellent credit. Senior scams are a very serious concern. I have seen people give away hundreds of thousands of dollars due to scams.

Sweepstakes mailings are very common and have been around for a long time. Some ask for cash to be sent by mail, and a senior may continue to receive mail indicating they are getting closer to the prize but need to send more money. I have witnessed many seniors continuing to send cash or a check thinking they are closer to the prize. I have one woman I help who keeps all her mail and has a folder of sweepstakes mailings. She writes notes on the envelope with the date and the amount of money she sent. When going through her mail, she told me to be careful because the checks being sent to her may be real. There was not one real check in there, but since they look real, she thought they were.

Mail scams also include requests for donations. The mail appears to be from a well-known charity. For example, mail from the American Heart & Stroke Association with a recognizable logo may request a donation to continue their cause. This would be easy to fall for. This fraudulent association looks familiar because it combined into one term the American

Heart Association and the American Stroke Association, each of which are legitimate associations.

Another scam is done through the internet. A pop-up window will appear indicating an anti-virus program needs to be installed immediately to protect the computer. Not only can these programs be expensive, but the creator can gain access to the computer and receive information that is dangerous in the wrong hands. I was with a client one day when she received a call from a man with a thick accent. He stated there was a security breech on her computer and he was calling to help her. He was wanting credit card information. She was confused by the call and was not sure how to respond. She did not even have a computer.

Phone scams can be performed numerous ways. One of the worst I have heard of is the "grandparent scam." The scammer will call the senior and say, "Hi Grandma/Grandpa, do you know who this is?" The grandparent says the name of the person they think it is. The scammer indicates they are in trouble and need money. Some scammers beg the grandparent to keep information from their parents because they are afraid of getting into trouble. These scammers may also call again using the name the grandparent gave and ask for more money. The "fake accident" scam is a similar scam. The senior receives a call stating their loved one was in a serious accident, is in the hospital, and needs money wired immediately to pay for emergency services. In my experience, the caller generally states the injured party is their grandchild. One story that sticks out in my mind is an elderly woman named Greta, who told me someone called when she was sleeping and said her grandchild was in a serious accident and needed money immediately. Greta said she was in a panic. Greta's daughter was the only child who had children, so she called her right away. In her panicked voice, she asked her daughter if one of the children were in trouble. Her daughter did not know of any issue, then Greta realized it was a scam. She received the same call a few nights later; she hung the phone up immediately. Greta did not have cognitive impairment, but the call was convincing enough to cause fright. Can you imagine getting a call like that in the middle of the night?

A common phone scam for people of all ages is the extended car-warranty scam. I receive these calls at least a couple of times a week. The caller states my car warranty has expired and I need to purchase a new warranty. They are usually calling about a vehicle I no longer own. I recently met with a client who fell for this scam. She purchased a car warranty on a car she has not owned in many years. The worst of phone scams is the funeral scam. In this scam, a widow is targeted through obituaries. The scammer will state the deceased had an outstanding debt.

There are many other scams that target the elderly. Collection scams claim there is a debt that is owed, and legal proceedings are threatened if payment is not received immediately. Door-to-door sales, predatory lending, and pyramid schemes can also occur but are not as common in the elderly. High-pressure sales tactics are easier to employ on an elderly person. There are also moving scams, in which items disappear or prices change from the negotiated rate and items are held until the new payment is made.

If your loved one has early dementia, it is important to monitor for scams and educate your loved one on precautions. Tips I provide to families to pass on to their loved ones include the following: do not give out personal information, do not give on impulse, never give cash, never sign a blank document, save mail that is suspicious and have someone else inspect it, take down call-back information from a suspicious caller, and do not wire or send money to someone who is not known.

When I have a client getting many scam calls, I advise family members to register the phone number on the National Do Not Call Registry. If mail seems to be an issue, you can have all mail forwarded to you. If there are financial concerns, I recommend replacing credit cards and checkbooks with a True Link card, which allows restrictions to protect the elderly from scams.

Increasing involvement in scams is often a warning sign of dementia as the areas of the brain that can identify a scam are altered. Additionally, with frontotemporal dementia, judgement is altered, making susceptibility even higher.

As William became more comfortable, I started to see him in his natural environment. I went to the home and found William sitting at the kitchen table in nothing but his underwear and shoes. In fact, he only wore underwear and shoes during all future visits. For being a man with means, I found his shoes to be surprising. They were worn and dirty. Donna indicated she has him wear his shoes in the shower for better grip. As a result, his shoes smelled horrible. I was not able to get rid of those shoes until we fitted him for orthotic shoes. He had a lot of pain with walking because of thin skin on the bottom of his feet, but the orthotic shoes made walking painless. Of course, in time, those shoes met the same fate.

Many of William's home visits were in his bedroom. He slept in the master bedroom, while Donna slept on a couch with the dogs. William often spit on the dresser and floor, so the area around his bed was dirty. During one visit, William wanted to show me some old items in his dresser. He pulled out pictures of half-dressed women who were not his wife. He told me about the women he dated while he was married to Donna. Donna was in the room, and she responded, "No locamente. I don't get involved." This is an example of the Donna-isms. Another common Donna-ism was, "I will be busy with all of the garbagio," when asked about her plans for the day. When the dogs would bark, she would say, "Behave a roo-roo." Occasionally I would hear her say, "I'm starving my brains out."

In the beginning I wondered where Donna was drinking and where the bottles were. There was no evidence she was actively drinking, except for the smell of alcohol. I came to learn she was a closet drinker, literally. She used the closet in the master bedroom to store wine and drink alcohol. On one visit, Donna said she needed to change her shirt prior to rushing into the closet and shutting the door. I heard bottles clinking together. Donna was in the closet for about twenty minutes. She came out wearing the exact same clothes. There will be more about Donna's closet drinking later.

I was managing William's doctor's appointments, which were numerous, at his insistence. At times, Donna came to the appointments, and I did my best to help her feel in control. She would make sure to have a few drinks before we would go, since it would be several hours before she could have another drink. We were at a cardiology appointment, waiting to be called back. It was five minutes past the time of the appointment, and Donna became irritated. She walked to the front desk and screamed at the receptionist. She said that it was unacceptable and that people were much more competent when she was younger. I apologized to the staff later. William was utterly embarrassed by her demeanor. We were called back to see the cardiologist. I provided an updated medication list. When the doctor reviewed it, he indicated William was taking quite a few medications. Donna said, "Yeah, he's a drug dealer." The room was quiet for a couple of seconds until I told the doctor William was not a drug dealer and indicated Donna was trying to be funny. Anytime Donna said she was coming along for a doctor's appointment, I had to brace myself for what was going to happen.

When William got agitated, he used foul language that upset his wife. One day we were talking about his niece, who was now acting as his decision maker. He was angry about Megan managing his money and felt she was an intrusion in his life. He said to me, "Next time Megan comes to my door, I am going to shoot her right in her face." I had a conversation with Megan and learned there were about twenty firearms in the home. During one of William's appointments that Donna also attended, Megan went into the home and removed the firearms. William would not have agreed to remove firearms from the home, in addition to the fact his dementia was advanced enough to pose an immediate risk. William was understandably angry about his firearms being removed without his permission, but it was necessary for everyone's safety.

### FIREARM SAFETY WITH DEMENTIA

Gun ownership in the United States is not uncommon. In fact, there are an estimated 393 million firearms in the United States, making the US the number one ranked country in the world for gun ownership.

In most situations, the presence of a gun does not create a problem. With dementia, there are changes in the brain, giving rise to the significant risk.

A common change with dementia and decreased memory is the struggle to recognize family and friends that were once familiar, creating the perception that an intruder is present. If any person perceives a threat, it would be reasonable to expect a firearm to be used for safety. Except with dementia, the perceived threat is not real and a loved one could be shot and even killed. Firearms also require complex cognitive abilities, including instinct in quick decision-making, which is compromised due to dementia. Additionally, behaviors consistent with dementia can include hallucinations and delusions, which would also pose a risk if a firearm were deemed by the person with dementia to be a necessary force.

In the earlier stages of dementia, it is important to have a conversation about firearm safety. A plan can be put into place to ensure safety for you and your loved ones. Separating from weapons can be difficult and should be done so with extreme caution. The first action to reduce risk is to lock or disable a gun or place guns in a safe place. This should be an immediate action, rather than a long-term action, as it does not fully ensure safety.

Determining placement of weapons can be allocated in several ways. A discussion about who should inherit firearms will allow the weapon to remain in the family. It can be suggested the firearm be turned over to the person determined to inherit the piece to continue upkeep. Another option is to sell valuable items to assist in paying for care. One may also elect to donate an antique firearm to a museum so that others can learn about the piece and appreciate it, just as your loved one has. While it is best for the person with dementia to plan what happens to their items, it is not necessary. If a firearm is present, a serious risk to others persists and removal of weapons against a person's wishes may be needed. When doing so, it is best to ensure the person with dementia is not home. Along with firearms, cases, ammunition, racks, and holsters should also be removed. Be mindful that anger and other emotions may occur because of the change. Be sympathetic to that emotion and support your loved one through the grief. If you need assistance in removing firearms, your local law enforcement may be able to help.

As William declined, the need for more equipment was needed. A hospital bed replaced his queen bed in his bedroom. He was angry about it, but Donna agreed with me and told him he needed it. William continued to fall and was not reporting his falls. I would find out about the fall because he would have an open wound. He fell in front of me one day after an appointment. I did my best to brace his fall onto the tiled floor, but he hit the floor hard. The fall caused a large skin tear to his arm. Because he could not get up and was losing a lot of blood, 911 was called . The paramedics bandaged his wound while I held his head in my arms. He refused to have further evaluation at the hospital. He was put into bed by the paramedics. There were many visits where he needed wound care, and Donna was always there to instruct me how to take care of his wounds. She told me to pour hydrogen peroxide on the wound and leave it open to air. Based on his wounds, her suggestion would not be best practice, so I educated her on how to properly care for a wound. I worked with his physicians to provide the best treatment. I would also irrigate his ears, as he would build up a lot of wax. One visit I was having difficulty getting ear wax out. Donna said she knew what to do. She brought me a metal tool with a sharp edge and told me to use it in his ear. I told her I would never do that because I could rupture his eardrum and that tool should never be used in someone's ears. She did not agree with me and wanted to show me how it can be used. I did not allow her to do so.

Even though William required a considerable amount of nursing care, I also tried to focus on quality of life. On one visit, I told him to get dressed because we were going to the park. He used to walk to the park every day before his stroke and meet friends along the way. He apparently also had a girlfriend at the park. Like Donna said, "No locamente." We sat in the park and he talked to me about his memories. He seemed to forget the negativity that took over his life. He enjoyed the breeze and watching children laugh and play. Driving back to his house, he saw one of his park friends. We pulled over and they talked for a bit. William was elated after that experience. That was one of the few moments of happiness I witnessed. On my next visit, William wanted to go to the park again. He was, of course, wearing his underwear and shoes. He grabbed his wallet and said, "Okay, let's go." I told him there was no way he was getting into my car like that. I had him get dressed and then we were on our way. He did not see his friends on any other park ride, but he was always hopeful he would see someone he knew and enjoyed driving around the park and reminiscing.

During one of the many appointments, we learned William had cataracts in both of his eyes that needed to be removed. William was scheduled for cataract surgery for his right eye, and the left was to be completed a week later. A caregiver brought him to the surgical center for the procedure. I received a call from the caregiver stating William was having chest pain. I told her to tell someone at the front desk to call 911. The building where he was going to have cataract surgery also had a medical clinic attached. An EKG was completed, and a physician confirmed William was having a heart attack. While waiting for the paramedics to arrive, the team at the clinic started CPR as William was non-responsive. He was taken to the hospital, and several hours after the first report of chest pain, I was told he was pronounced dead after attempts to resuscitate.

I spoke to Megan and we decided it would be best to go to Donna's home and let her know what happened in person. Donna answered the door and appeared confused. She looked around the outside area and asked where William was. We sat her down and told her he had a massive heart attack and did not survive. Donna was very quiet and expressionless. I am not sure if Donna expected his time was limited or if she grieved quietly, but I never saw her mourn the death of her husband.

William did not want a memorial service or any real recognition of his death. Donna was taken to the funeral home several days after William's death. She went into a backroom on her own to say her goodbyes. From my understanding, William was not in a coffin, but rather a basic box and would later be taken for cremation. Donna was in the back for a couple of minutes, came out, and was ready to go home. She had a blank stare on her face and not one tear. I know she drank quite a bit before we went to the funeral home, and I think her intoxication helped her feel devoid of emotion for that moment. Donna was taken home and her new life without William began.

# CHAPTER 9:
# A NEW BEGINNING

Death is not a failure of medical science
but the last act of life.

—Patch Adams, MD

Donna's cognitive impairment secondary to alcoholism had been monitored while William was alive. With William's death, a new plan was needed to ensure Donna was safe. Twenty-four-hour care had been put into place to monitor William after his cataract surgery. Megan wanted to keep the twenty-four-hour care in place to monitor and provide support. Along with that, Megan wanted me to manage Donna's care. As with Shirley's situation, the increased care gave us a better perspective in how Donna was functioning throughout the day.

During the initial period after William's death, the caregivers reported Donna was sleeping very little. Even with the master bedroom being empty, Donna continued to sleep on the couch with the dogs. She woke up every couple of hours, went into the closet in the master bedroom, then back to the couch to sleep. Donna stated that she was not concerned about her sleeping pattern because she has always been a light sleeper. I suspected Donna had withdrawals just hours after her last drink. The caregivers also noticed Donna ate very little food. Most of her calories were coming from alcohol.

Speaking of food, I wanted to evaluate the contents of her refrigerator and pantry. It is common for people with cognitive impairment to have food in the kitchen that should not be consumed. Most of the food and fluids in her refrigerator and pantry were expired, and not by a few days but a few years. The refrigerator drawers contained rotten produce that liquefied and coated the bottom of the drawers. Donna had milk that was curdled, and I could barely stand the smell as I emptied the bottle. In that moment, my mind flashed to William. He had difficulty eating the food that was prepared for him and most likely it was because the food was spoiled. Since Donna insisted on doing everything herself, cleaning her refrigerator was done when she was not around. The best time to clean was when she went into the closet.

The general cleanliness of the house was also a concern. Donna would not allow caregivers to clean and would insist it is on her list of things to do. Donna's closet time allowed the initiation of cleaning, which she usually allowed if it had already been started. The couch covers were coated with dirt and dog hair. One day while she was in the closet,

I removed the couch covers and put them in the washer. When she came out of the closet, she asked where the covers were, and I stated, "You put them in the washer." She would acknowledge she did so in attempts to avoid appearing forgetful. Another time I tried to wash the couch covers, she came out of the closet quicker than normal, so I threw them behind the couch, but they were still visible if she came around the corner. She noticed the covers were missing and then saw the covers on the floor. She asked what happened. I told her she took them off and was going to put them in the washer. She said, "Oh, yeah," picked them up and put them in the washer. This tactic is another example of therapeutic fibbing.

**HOME SAFETY**

Housekeeping and general hygiene generally become an issue as dementia progresses. A person with dementia will likely cease home maintenance and general housekeeping. These issues demonstrate a progression of the illness. When aiding, extreme caution should be taken, as to allow what is necessary without causing undue stress or agitation. It is also important to maintain optimal home safety. Home areas I assess include the following:

**Bathroom**

- Presence of grab bars as well as stability and placement of grab bars

- Is the surface of the floor and the shower nonskid?
- A raised toilet seat may be needed if sitting down becomes an issue
- Water faucet temperature should be clearly labeled
- The water heater should be set no higher than 120 degrees
- Nightlights are present

**Kitchen**

- Emergency phone numbers should be listed on the refrigerator
- Dishes should be stored on lower shelves and easy to get to
- Towels and curtains should be kept away from the stove
- Off indicators on the stove and appliances should be clearly marked (there are also auto shutoff devices for the stove if there are concerns it is left on)
- Plastic containers and dishes are preferred over glassware
- Cleaning products are clearly labeled
- Pots and pans are lightweight and in good working order
- Fire extinguisher is present, within reach of the stove, and in good working order

**Electrical**

- Condition of electrical appliances, such as cords and plugs, are checked regularly; wiring must be insulated
- Electric outlets are ground fault interrupter (GFI) protected and are functioning correctly
- Circuits and extension cords are not overloaded
- Electric cords are in good working order and are tucked away
- Electric heaters are away from curtains, rugs, and furnishings

**General**

- Adequate lighting throughout the house is important
- The occupant should be able to identify two ways to get out of the home during an emergency
- The home, including paint, walls, and outside area, is in good working order
- Fall hazards are removed, which includes throw rugs, cluttered spaces, and cords
- First-aid kit is available and has adequate supplies
- Fire alarm system is in good working order

If you are providing housekeeping to your loved one, you want to do so in a manner that is nonjudgmental and without the perception of inability on your loved one's part. Hiring a housekeeper may be appropriate, but this should also be considered with caution as a person with dementia is more likely to be taken advantage of. It is necessary to evaluate the contents of the refrigerator and pantry. Going through someone's refrigerator without consent can be offensive, so it must be done in a thoughtful manner. In some cases, you can go through the refrigerator with the person with dementia and allow them to be a part of the process. Often, this causes more anxiety. It is usually best to clean the refrigerator when the person with dementia is not present. Usually, the person with dementia does not notice items missing from the refrigerator, but surprises can be anticipated.

One of my clients with middle-stage Alzheimer's was struggling in her home environment. She had a housekeeper who she was very familiar with, so the cleanliness of the home was not an issue. The housekeeper was not responsible for contents in the refrigerator. My client was experiencing diarrhea on a regular basis, without any clear indication of the cause. The first time I investigated her refrigerator and pantry, I knew the cause. There were items that had been expired for nearly ten years. Vegetables and fruits were liquified and covered in mold. There was very little food that was edible. I thought cleaning her refrigerator would be a good first step and then regular maintenance would be simple. I threw away a large amount of food from her refrigerator and pantry; she did not notice when she went into the kitchen. The next day, however, she had me follow her to the garbage cans to take notice of her project. There were cans and boxes against the wall and food from the refrigerator on top of the recycle trash can. She indicated that someone threw her food away and that most of the food was completely fine. She brought the foods she thought were still good back into the house. I was taken aback by this, but knew my method was not going to work with her. I now visit when she is out of the home with her caregiver, pull out expired and spoiled items from her refrigerator and pantry, bag it up, and take it home with me for disposal. I move items around in her refrigerator and pantry so that there do not appear to be empty spaces and she does not notice there are missing items. I have learned over the course of my career one method is not right for everyone. I must be observant and flexible to adjust my methods for the good of my clients.

I was intrigued by Donna's ability to hide bottles and wondered what her process was. I was covering a shift one day and got to experience her procedure. Donna transferred empty wine bottles into an ice chest in her garage. I witnessed her, from a distance, moving wine bottles from the ice chest into a linen shopping bag. Donna indicated she was going to the grocery store. She declined a ride and indicated she wanted to walk by herself. Donna walked down the street and then down into an alleyway behind neighboring homes. I observed her transferring the wine bottles from her linen bag into someone else's garbage can. She looked over both shoulders before doing so but did not have an awareness I was watching. She continued walking down the alleyway with her empty linen bag and presumably to the grocery store. Donna came through the front door with her linen bag and additional plastic bags with groceries. She left the plastic bags at the door and immediately brought the linen bag to the closet. The linen bag would remain in the closet and was used to transport empty bottles to the ice chest.

## ALCOHOL USE WITH DEMENTIA

While it is known excessive alcohol use can cause damage to the brain and increase the risk of Alzheimer's disease and other forms of dementia, there is little discussion about the effects of alcohol when dementia is already present. It goes without saying, alcohol use of any kind when cognitive impairment is present leads to increased symptoms associated with dementia. Physicians advise those with dementia to avoid drinking altogether, but this direction is not simple. Alcohol use can be habitual, and with decreased judgment due to dementia, habitual drinking can lead to excessive alcohol use, even if an alcohol abuse has not previously been an issue.

I have a client who was living alone without caregiver support and was accustomed to having alcoholic drinks with her husband every night prior to his death. She continued to consume alcohol but seemed to consume more and was losing control of herself. She was injuring herself frequently and was not seeking medical care when she was injured. Her daughter implemented caregiving services to keep her safe, but she continued to drink when alone. Shortly after becoming involved, we switched out her alcoholic beverages with non-alcoholic substitutes. She did not seem to notice. When going to the store, we would switch wine and beer with non-alcoholic versions, and she did not notice this either. When the switch was made, there was a very noticeable positive impact on her cognition. Although she had dementia, which is progressive, she was much more intact and improving despite her diagnosis. Eventually she did begin to decline but continued to drink non-alcoholic beverages without an awareness she was no longer drinking alcohol. With her decline, she rarely went to the grocery store. I started to pick up her drinks, and along with the caregivers, we were able to place beverages in areas she was accustomed. The caregivers served a non-alcoholic beer with dinner, which she enjoyed. It provided her with quality of life, without the negative cognitive effects.

There are many options for non-alcoholic beverages, such as wine, beer, gin, whiskey, and tequila. If your loved one has a favorite brand, you could refill the bottle with the non-alcoholic version of their favorite drink. Some families choose to allow their loved one an alcoholic drink on occasion.

Donna had many interesting stories, which always displayed her as the hero or as a sacred one. The first of these stories involved a time her and William went camping. They were in the woods and a large bear appeared with her baby cub. Donna states the bear appeared to be in protection mode, so she was concerned the bear would attack them. Donna told the bear everything was okay and held out her hand to shake the bear's hand. The bear shook her hand, turned around, and waved as she walked off with her cub. Another story took place when she lived in Hawaii and was on the surfing scene. She told me that she was the only "chick" out there and that the guys thought she did not belong. One day she spotted a great white shark. Everyone got out of the water and were on the shore, terrified. Donna told the shark he was scaring everyone and needed to go away. The shark raised a fin in the air to wave at her and swam away. There were variations to these stories, and sometimes the animals verbally communicated with her. She had a pet snake as a small child and used to walk it on a leash around the neighborhood. She had a large Dutch rabbit, a Great Dane, and a burro. She was the only one in her family that could care for these animals, and they only wanted to be with her. I would listen to her stories and tell her how amazing she was, and she had a great sense of pride. I figured with everything else going on in her life, she could at least feel she had some importance in this world.

Part of my role with Donna was to get appropriate medical care in place and ensure her needs were met. Because she was resistant to doctor's appointments for herself, I brought in a mobile physician. Donna appeared to enjoy the visits from Dr. Cohen but would try to cancel the visit prior to it occurring. I told her about the appointments shortly before he was coming to ensure compliance. This is important for anyone with dementia. Often when a person with dementia is told of an appointment with too much notice, anxiety increases followed by many questions. It is best to tell a person with dementia about an appointment several hours— at the most—before the appointment. I was always present for these appointments so that I could ensure her provider was receiving accurate information about Donna's medical condition and her continued drinking patterns. When the doctor asked Donna how much she drinks a day, she stated she may have a couple of glasses of wine per week. I asked Donna how she knows how many glasses she drinks, since from all appearances, I suspected she drank straight from the bottle. She simply indicated she pours wine into a wine glass. I then asked her if she has wine glasses in the closet. She did not have an answer and was shocked, as though she did not have an awareness anyone knew her secret.

Once Donna became more comfortable with medical care, I was able to move forward with more specific care related to alcoholism and suspected liver damage. Donna saw a gastroenterologist to determine the extent of damage to her liver. Per physician orders, I took Donna to an imaging center to have an abdominal ultrasound completed. She waited about five minutes and then became angry she was still waiting. I felt like I had a flashback of the time we went to William's cardiology appointment. Donna attempted to reschedule the appointment and I was doing my best to distract her. With a lot of convincing, Donna completed the ultrasound. We went back to the gastroenterologist, who gave Donna a diagnosis of alcoholic cirrhosis of the liver. With cirrhosis, the normal functioning of the liver is altered. As a result, Donna was at a higher risk of bleeding, peritoneal infections, ascites (swelling of the abdomen), encephalopathy, liver cancer, and potential for damage to other organs. Common symptoms seen with cirrhosis also include weakness, decreased appetite, jaundice (yellowing of the skin), itching, easy bruising, and fatigue. The gastroenterologist asked Donna about her drinking. She stated she had a couple glasses of wine a week. She was obviously impaired and smelled of alcohol, so the gastroenterologist knew unequivocally she was not being truthful. The doctor told Donna he could not do anything for her if she is actively drinking. The doctor refused to provide any treatment, monitoring, or support while Donna continued to drink.

Donna continued to receive medical services in the home. Beacuse of her diagnosis of cirrhosis, Dr. Cohen started her on medication to minimize damage to the liver and supplements to replace deficits due to chronic alcoholism. Donna was not one for medication and compliance was challenging. It was not until she suffered more serious consequences of cirrhosis that she agreed to take medication. She was building up fluid in the abdomen and she was not able to button her pants. She reverted to sweatpants. She started wearing a wool coat around the house in attempt to cover up her increased abdominal girth. This was followed with swelling in her legs, ankles, and feet. Her legs were probably triple their normal size. Eventually the skin on her legs opened and fluid started to leak from the openings. Donna agreed to take a diuretic to decrease fluid buildup, and with that, she accepted the other medications for her liver.

Donna's niece, Megan, needed to get an inventory of items in the home, so I was tasked with getting her out of the home. I scheduled an appointment for Donna to get a manicure and pedicure. I was concerned with her being out of the home for more than a few hours because I suspected she would start withdrawal from alcohol. With Megan's permission, I purchased a four pack of small bottles of wine. Toward the end of Donna's service, withdrawal symptoms were apparent. Donna became very anxious and started to sweat. She said she needed to go home immediately. I wanted to get her out of the salon without causing any embarrassment to Donna. Walking to the car she was shaking and sweat was dripping down her face. Once she was in the car, I provided a small bottle of wine. I never witnessed Donna drinking until that day. Her need to alleviate withdrawal symptoms was far greater than her determination to convince others she does not consume alcohol. She drank the small bottle of wine quickly and then had another. Her symptoms improved immediately. I then knew she started withdrawal only two hours after her last drink. I also came to realize why she could only sleep for a few hours at time. My heart hurt for her. I cannot imagine all the pain she felt and the pain that led her down this road.

Donna continued the same path until one day, right around Christmas, I received a call from the caregiver indicating there was blood all over the bathroom floor. Donna stated it was just a couple of drops. The caregiver sent a picture of the bathroom; it appeared like her bathroom was a murder scene. There was blood splattered on the walls, blood smears on the tile, and puddles of blood on the floor. Donna stated she did not need any treatment and stated the problem would go away on its own. She was eventually sent to the hospital. We learned she had a gastrointestinal bleed and esophageal varices. Her blood was thin from her liver dysfunction. It was as if someone pulled the rug from under her.

Donna had many complications while in the hospital, requiring tests and procedures, such as a paracentesis. Donna was in the hospital for several weeks before being sent to a rehabilitation center to gain strength since she had not walked during her hospitalization. Donna was not able to walk on her own and was needing significant assistance. Donna was resistant to care and would not participate in therapy. The rehabilitation facility had to discharge Donna because she was not participating. Donna was placed in an assisted living group home to receive care and oversight.

Upon arriving at the group home, it was apparent Donna's health was deteriorating. At 5'6" she was down to ninety pounds. She was confined to a bed and was sleeping most of the time. She did not have interest in food and was eating very little. A hospice evaluation was completed, and hospice services were started at the group home. The admission nurse for hospice indicated she thought Donna was within days of death. Several weeks later, Donna perked up a bit. Donna was able to transfer with assistance to a wheelchair and was starting to eat a little more. She was able to stay awake for longer periods of time. It had been about two months since her last drink of alcohol. As time went on, she appeared to improve, and she was taken off hospice services. She started talking in sentences again and even engaged in some cognitive activities. One day I went to the group home to visit her and she was walking in the hallway. I had to do a double take because I could not believe she was walking. It had been months since she last walked. I remember telling Megan that her walking was a good thing and a bad thing. We were thrilled she was improving, but she was unstable on her feet. Donna did receive physical therapy and continued to gain strength. She did need to be monitored constantly when walking, which seemed feasible at the group home where she was residing.

I went to visit her one day and found her in the wheelchair at the dining table with a chair diagonal to the wall, preventing her from having space to stand up. Being trapped in that position and wanting to get up, she would put as much force as possible on her arms to try to get up. She had large skin tears on both of her arms; she literally had no skin over some areas. She would also kick her legs and had skin tears on her shins. The group home manager said it was necessary to keep her in the wheelchair to keep her from falling. Despite education on the use of restraints, the group home manager continued to restrain Donna in the wheelchair. For her safety and quality of life, it was necessary for Donna to move to another group home.

## RESTRAINTS

Physical restraints are used seemingly to protect a person with dementia; however, they are seldom effective and often harmful. A restraint can be delivered by a variety of methods. A physical restraint can be carried out by trapping or isolating a person, such as in Donna's situation. Physical restraints can be items placed on a person to hold them in place, such as restraints tied to the wrist and then tied to a bed. Physical restraints are also recognized by any apparatus used to restrict movement or prevent a person from leaving. This can include bed rails on a hospital bed, a tray on a chair that is not used for eating or activity, or putting medical equipment by the bed to fill in empty spaces around the bed.

There are situations where restraints are necessary. For example, when working in the ICU, I had patients who were on a ventilator. Although they were sedated, there were times where the patient started to come out of a state of sedation. Some patients woke up enough to be able to pull on the tube going down their throat. Patients on a ventilator had restraints on their wrists to prevent them from pulling the tube out if they wake up. It would be a natural reaction to try to pull a tube out of your throat but doing so causes harm, so the restraint is necessary to prevent harm. There are many protocols in place when restraints are used to ensure the skin on the wrist is not damaged or the vascularization is not affected.

Restraints can also be chemical, meaning a chemical is provided, causing lethargy and preventing a behavior or ability to escape. With dementia, medications may be needed if other interventions are not successful and the person with dementia is a risk to themselves or others. Restraints of any kind are uncommon and should be used with extreme caution.

The use of physical restraints with a person with cognitive impairment is almost always unacceptable. A person with dementia may try to walk when weak and need support to do so safely. A person with dementia may act out by hitting or kicking and need support that tries to understand there is a reason for the behavior, helping to alleviate whatever discomfort is causing that behavior. A person with dementia may have exit-seeking behaviors and try to leave the home unattended and need support to find distraction and feel safe. Can you imagine being confused about where you are, feeling discomfort and not knowing how to communicate that, and being tied to a chair? Imagine the fear you would feel. I always recommend stepping into the shoes of the person with dementia and thinking of how it would feel if you were in that position. The right answer should always come to you.

The new assisted living group home was supportive of Donna's need to ambulate and gain independence. She was soon walking on her own and gradually became more independent. There was another gentleman in the home who took a liking to Donna. They spent a great deal of time together. They would hold hands, sing together, watch television, and go outside for walks together. The social interaction was helpful in building upon the skills in her search for independence. Donna started to shower and groom herself and was able to take care of her personal care needs.

For some time, evidence of cirrhosis lingered, although Donna's health seemed to be improving. She was required to have an esophagogastroduodenoscopy (EGD) every six months. In this procedure, a camera is inserted into the mouth and down the upper part of the gastrointestinal system to search for any dilated blood vessels that can lead to bleeding. When Donna first started having this procedure, bands were placed over dilated blood vessels, but as time went on, she did not have dilated blood vessels anymore. She eventually was able to get an EGD every two years. Donna's labs were abnormal, showing damage to the liver function, but as time went on, her labs completely normalized. She continued to receive abdominal ultrasounds every six months, which showed an enlarged liver but no indication of cancerous growths. Donna had been sober for three years when her liver showed normalization. Unfortunately, the damage her brain experienced from chronic alcoholism is not reversible. The condition Donna experienced is known as Wernicke-Korsakoff syndrome.

## DEMENTIA: KORSAKOFF SYNDROME

Korsakoff syndrome is a chronic memory disorder caused by a severe thiamine (vitamin B-1) deficiency. Thiamine deficiency affects several biochemicals that allow signals to transmit among brain cells. Eventually, the deficiency destroys brain cells and causes microscopic bleeding and scar tissue. Most of the time, Korsakoff syndrome is caused by alcohol abuse, although there are other causes for the disorder, such as cancer, malabsorption of nutrients, and chronic infections. Thiamine converts sugar to energy in the brain cells. When thiamine levels are low, the brain cannot generate enough energy to function properly. Korsakoff syndrome is generally preceded by Wernicke encephalopathy, which is an acute condition due to severe thiamine deficiency. Wernicke encephalopathy causes confusion, lack of coordination, involuntary movements, and disruption to the brain.

Korsakoff syndrome is believed to be less common than Alzheimer's disease, vascular dementia, frontotemporal dementia, and Lewy body dementia; however, there is the possibility it is not diagnosed appropriately, making the prevalence lower than actual occurrence. A common symptom of Korsakoff syndrome is memory impairment, which can include difficulty learning new information and difficulty recalling short- and long-term memories. A fascinating common symptom of Korsakoff syndrome is confabulation, in which the person fabricates detailed stories to fill in gaps in memory. As you may recall, Donna told many seemingly fabricated stories about animals communicating with her. Once Wernicke encephalopathy is corrected, confusion will start to clear, but the underlying Korsakoff syndrome may present with long-term memory problems that are not reversible.

In Donna's case, memory impairment was evident; however, it was difficult to ascertain if the impairment was related to encephalopathy or the constant presence of alcohol in her system. After her acute episode, the absence of alcohol and treatment with thiamine did stabilize her, but her continued memory impairment persisted. Donna's overall prognosis is good, but she will always have memory impairment from Korsakoff syndrome. Considering her age, it is unfortunate she is not able to live the rest of her life freely and independently. She will require monitoring and assistance with IADLs for the rest of her life.

# Chapter 10:
# Taking Care of You

Have patience with all things, but chiefly have
patience with yourself. Do not lose courage in considering your own imperfections, but instantly set about
remedying them, every day a task anew.

—St. Francis DeSales

To say caring for a person with dementia is a challenge is
an understatement. I have witnessed many family members
and health-care professionals feel burnout, especially if all
their efforts are going into caring for a person with dementia
while neglecting their own needs. Studies show that caregivers of people with dementia have suppressed immune
systems, increased rates of infection, and a higher prevalence of depression. Around 40–70 percent of caregivers
have clinically significant signs of depression, and 25–50
percent of these individuals meet the diagnostic criteria for
major depression.

There are many emotions you will feel through the caregiving process, and you may struggle with some of those feelings. Many people who are caring for someone with dementia feel conflicting emotions at the same time. For example, a daughter may feel anger when behaviors are occurring, but feel guilty for screaming out of anger. Anticipatory grief is also very common, which is the process of grieving in anticipation of a loss. I remember speaking to the daughter of a client with late-stage dementia about grieving each loss along the process, such as the loss of the ability to walk or talk. Each loss felt like another piece of her mother was taken away. She grieved while her mother was alive. While feeling this grief she also felt guilty because she hoped her mom would die so that her mother would not suffer anymore. I have heard of family members stating they did not really grieve after the death because they went through the grieving process while their loved one was alive.

## CARING FOR A SPOUSE WITH DEMENTIA

The dynamics of a marriage can change drastically when dementia is present in one of the spouses. A spouse may initially be providing reminders and ensuring safety, but as time progresses, a spouse will be providing more care, both physically and emotionally. Maintaining an emotional connection can be difficult when you are also assisting in the bathroom, providing shower assistance, and helping with grooming. Although some aspects of your relationship will change, there are ways to maintain an enriching relationship with your spouse. Holding hands, hugging, and listening to music together can help maintain a closeness. If you had a routine with your spouse, try to keep that routine if it is feasible. Allowing your spouse as much independence as possible is essential.

There will be times you will be frustrated and even angry. You will need to set new expectations for yourself and your relationship. Ask for help if you need a break. If you have children in the area or even close friends who are willing to help, allow the help. This is hard for many spouses, but if you do not take care of yourself, your spouse will suffer in the long run. Taking care of yourself includes following up with doctors for any medical conditions you may have. You will need methods to reduce your stress, whether it is having a spa day or sitting alone in the wilderness, it is important to maintain your emotional health.

A common issue I have heard from married couples learning to live with dementia is the loss of social interactions. Many times, family friends become distant and are not sure how to be a part of your new life. I find that people who have not experienced caring for someone with dementia fear the unknown and do not want to complicate your life any more than it is. Early in the diagnosis, it is important to let your close friends know what is going on and educate them on how to be present with your spouse. If you and your spouse used to have dinner parties, perhaps have dinner with one couple at a time so that your friends can interact and build a comfort level. Letting your friends know what to expect and how to handle situations can ease their fear. Encourage your friends to spend time with your spouse. For example, if your spouse and a friend enjoyed watching football together, ask his friend to come over, which would allow you some time to be alone or run errands. Your friends do not become distant because they do not want the burden; they become distant because they do not know any other way to be.

## Parenting Your Parents

A common strain expressed by the children of a person with dementia is the concept of role reversal. When a person with dementia is no longer capable of making good decisions, their children will need to step in to help with decisions and management of daily life. Children express feeling like their parent's parent. Additionally, many children caring for a parent with dementia are in the sandwich generation, meaning they are also working and raising a family of their own. While some children are firm with their parents and initiate care that is needed, most children are conflicted with the change in the relationship and their awareness of the need to make their parents safe.

The term *parenting your parents* is intended not to construct the idea that your parents are children or that you are their dictator but rather to depict the emotional struggle that many children have when they begin to provide more care for their parents. If your parent has been diagnosed with dementia, being proactive is more beneficial in the long run. Many families wait for a crisis, which alters the decision-making process and does not allow proper time to research options. You should start conversations with your parent early and involve your parent in the decision-making process. Knowing your parent's desires while having the ability to express wishes allows you a better opportunity to align your decisions with their wants and needs. Additionally, promising a parent to stay home forever is discouraged as it may not be feasible. Although the promise is well intended, you do not know what the future will hold for your parent.

It is also common for the adult child to have suspicions of altered cognition, but their significant other is covering deficits. For example, I cared for a woman whose husband recently passed away. Her daughter suspected memory impairment. When her father passed away and she stepped in to help her mom, she came to find out her mom had a diagnosis of dementia and her dad was helping her keep it a secret between the two of them. I have observed spouses and significant others go to great lengths to keep the diagnosis and their struggles a secret.

I encourage children to engage a care manager early to allow the care manager time to build a rapport and understand your parent's baseline. A care manager can be proactive with care needs and can assist during moments of crisis. Often, a parent fails to listen to their child but may be receptive to suggestions from a non-family member. A care manager can also provide guidance and support throughout the disease progression. I also encourage children to ensure legal documents are in place. An elder law attorney will be a useful resource initially and as financial situations change. An elder law attorney can also protect assets and help you understand what your parent may be entitled to for ongoing care needs.

It is exceptionally difficult when roles are reversed and you may be afraid to make certain decisions because you do not want to upset your parent. It is important to remember your parent lacks the ability to advocate for themselves. If your parent is making good decisions, allow those decisions. Your parent wants to feel in control and a part of the process. It is helpful to make suggestions in a way that sounds like it is your parent's idea. Your parent most likely will push back at times. If a parent is making bad decisions that could lead to serious consequences, you must look past their anger and remind yourself you are acting in their best interest.

I have consulted with many adult children who are the primary caregiver and whose siblings are minimally involved. If you are in this situation, you may feel resentment toward your siblings. I have heard of distant siblings calling and directing the child performing the care without understanding the situation or what the care needs are. I was consulting with a woman who was caring for her mother, and I listened to her grievances about the process. She said she was the only one out of four children who stepped up. She moved her mother into her home to care for her. Her brother would call and state their mom does not have dementia and their mother needs to be cared for in a better way. Her brother never offered to take their mother for the weekend. Her other two siblings were distant, out of fear of the disease and had no interest in learning about dementia. This can be frustrating and upsetting. You must remember you are doing the best you can do. If you have a sibling providing most of the care for a parent, get involved and work with your sibling to lessen the burden. This is a time family should be coming together, not splitting apart.

## DEMENTIA CARE WHEN YOU ARE NOT THE ADULT CHILD OR SPOUSE

Although the primary caregiver is usually an adult child or a spouse, there are many other familial situations where you may be caring for a person with dementia. I have a client whose niece is the caregiver. I have heard of a cousin providing care and even a former spouse. There are even times when a younger child is growing up in a home with a parent with early onset dementia or a grandparent who was moved in to receive more help. Any of these situations can present with similar and different challenges. Regardless of the connection, the relationship will be strained in a way that requires you to pivot.

I find it particularly challenging when a child is raised in a home with a person with dementia. The child may be required to "watch grandma" for a couple of hours to make sure she does not wander. This can be scary and confusing to a younger child. The brain of a child is not fully formed until the early twenties, and the ability to problem solve is not well developed. If the child has a parent with early onset dementia, the nature of their entire relationship can be affected. If you have a child in the home, in addition to a person with dementia, it is important to educate the child on dementia and how to respond. The child will also need opportunities for self-care. Ensure the child's mental and emotional health are also considered.

I have also encountered situations where a neighbor or old friend is providing care, or at a minimum, is serving as the power of attorney. Even if there is not an emotional connection, some decisions can take a toll on the person who has stepped in to help. In many cases, the person who has stepped in knows very little about dementia and does what they believe to be right.

## Plan for the Future

At some point, most caregivers supporting a person with dementia will require additional assistance. There are many options to consider based on the goals of yourself and the person with dementia. If possible, options should be discussed with your loved one so that they can be as involved in their future as much as possible.

## CARE IN THE COMMUNITY

Some people hire a caregiver to spend time with their loved one while they run errands, get respite, or even go to work. There are many considerations when hiring a caregiver. States have different laws on how caregivers are regulated. It is important to know the standards in your state to ensure your loved one is getting proper care. Some states do not have any standards of care, so your due diligence will be mandatory.

There are many agencies that provide caregivers and nursing assistants. The benefit of using an agency is that they are responsible for liability and other necessary insurance, background checks, and bonding of their employees. An agency takes out taxes and issues payment, instead of you being responsible to pay the caregiver. If the caregiver provided substandard care or performed inappropriately, the agency is responsible for disciplinary action, which could include reporting to law enforcement. If the caregiver is out sick, the agency will identify a suitable replacement.

Some people hire a private caregiver; however, use extreme caution if you want to take this route. Generally, a private caregiver does not carry insurances an agency would cover, so if they are injured on the job, you may be responsible for health-care costs. Also, you are their boss, so if they need time off, you will be required to find a replacement. Private caregivers do not usually take taxes out of the money you pay them, so you will need to set up a system to legally provide payment to the caregiver. An agency will cost more than a private caregiver, but there are layers of protection for you and your loved one. A private caregiver may cost substantially less than hiring an agency. If you do decide to use a private caregiver, ensure there are expectations for the care of your loved one and assistance in the home. You should perform a background check periodically as well. You will want to make sure you have a system for paying the caregiver and ensure you have proper insurance to cover any potential issues.

Another care option is an adult day center. Centers provide a planned program and can vary greatly regarding services provided, level of care, availability, health monitoring, and activities. When researching for a day program, it is important to ensure the center can provide specialized care for a person with dementia. Prior to visiting a center, have a list of questions you want to ask to make sure the program is best suited for your loved one's needs. Some questions include the following:

- What assistance is provided? Some programs assist with toileting, transfers, bathing, administering medication, and checking vital signs. Some centers also have access to physical or occupational therapy services.
- Can the center provide services for a person with dementia that has behaviors? What is their capacity to manage behaviors? When is it determined if

behaviors exclude your loved one from attending the program?

- What supplementary services are offered? If the center does provide additional services, inquire how much that service costs and what the service entails. Some centers provide transportation to and from, which is attractive for a caregiver who is still working. Some centers also offer medical services from a mobile provider, as well as haircuts, manicures, and other beauty services.

- Are meals and/or snacks provided? Ask to see their menu. Find out if they make accommodations for special diets or food intolerances. Does the center feed the attendees if they are not able to feed themselves? Is there a cost for meals and snacks?

- What activities are provided? Ask to see their calendar of activities. It would be helpful to be present during an activity to observe how the center gets attendees to participate.

- What is the staffing ratio? What kind of training is provided?

- Is the center accredited, licensed, or certified? If applicable, ask to see the state survey to ensure the center complies with the Department of Health. Rules on these aspects vary by state.

- What are the days and hours of operation? What happens if you are late to pick up your loved one?

- Is there a maximum level of care the center can provide? When considering a center, you want to make sure they can provide increased care if your loved one needs it in the future.

- What is the fee schedule? Are the prices inclusive of all services, or some? If not all, what are the costs of additional services? Is financial assistance available if needed? Does the center assist in the process of using state assistance if applicable?
- Does the center complete and review a care plan? What is the process for that?

I recommend visiting the center a couple of times at different times of the day. Try the food to see if the food would be pleasing to your loved one. Talk to other participants and/or ask for references from the center. Some people with dementia enjoy the program from the beginning and some will state they do not want to return. It is best to allow your loved one several attempts before deciding if you will discontinue the program. Often, once a person goes to the program more and becomes more comfortable, there is enjoyment in going. This can be beneficial to you and your loved one. Adult day centers can be used in conjunction with home caregiving services as well.

## CARE IN A FACILITY

Hiring a caregiver can be costly and may not even be a feasible living arrangement for you and your loved one. Some people with dementia move into a facility setting. There are many setting options for your loved one to consider. A

CCRC was mentioned previously, which includes a variety of services on one campus to provide every level of care needed throughout the aging process. It is advisable if you are considering a CCRC to visit all the levels of care before deciding. I have worked with clients who did not like the skilled nursing unit or the memory-care unit and moved to the community because of the independent living (IL) options. You should feel comfortable with all levels of care before making the move into a CCRC. Additionally, many require money upfront, which can be a significant amount of money, and this option may not be financially viable for your loved one. If that is the case, it is important to move into a setting that is currently suitable and can provide more care as the need arises. Your loved one may need to move if their level-of-care need surpasses what can be provided, which should be avoided if possible.

IL is an option for seniors who are still independent in their care but prefer a smaller living environment with amenities suitable for their needs. Apartment sizes can vary. IL services may include fitness rooms and classes, swimming pools, dining rooms, cafes, bars, a library, a wellness center, and a spa. Many also include housekeeping services. For a person with dementia requiring supervision, IL would not be a suitable option, as it would not be a long-term viable option, unless it is coupled with caregiving services.

Assisted living (AL) is a level of care between IL and nursing home care. The resident has the personal space of an apartment but also has many services to assist in daily care. The apartments are generally smaller than an IL apartment and may include a kitchenette instead of a full kitchen. Some AL facilities have nursing services around the clock, while others have limited nursing services. A resident in AL would need to be independent enough to be alone safely in their apartment. There is a pendant service for residents to use in the event they need help in their apartment, but your loved one would require awareness of the need to ask for help and would have to understand to press the button if needed. AL facilities have a dining room, which offers three meals a day. Snacks and fluids are also provided during the day. AL also provides medication management and assistance with activities of daily living, such as showering and dressing. AL also has activities available throughout the day, and some also have outings at a regular interval.

A skilled nursing facility (SNF) provides advanced care on a temporary or permanent basis. Your loved one may need intermittent SNF placement if there was a hospitalization and intense care is needed. Medicare Part A covers skilled nursing care under the guidance of the Centers for Medicare and Medicaid Services. A SNF provides nursing services, as well as nursing assistants and physical, occupational, and speech therapy. There are some people with dementia that remain in a SNF on a permanent basis due to extensive health-care needs in addition to dementia.

Memory-care units can be a part of a senior living community or as its own entity and are intended for people with cognitive impairment. Staff encompass skills to provide personal care services, as well as skills specific to caring for people with cognitive impairment. AL and SNF may have staff that understand the needs of someone with dementia, but often, they are not equipped to manage the complex needs like a memory-care unit can. One key benefit of a memory-care unit is the safety feature of locked doors that can only be opened by staff. Memory-care units cater to the needs of any stage of dementia, up to and including the end of life. In the absence of needs that require skilled nursing services, a person with dementia can remain in a memory-care unit and end-of-life care can be provided by staff, with the support of hospice, if desired. Memory-care units provide activities that are suitable for people with cognitive impairment. There are usually other services like access to a beauty salon. Staff encourage the person with dementia to do as much as safely possible, while eventually providing more assistance, including total care when the time comes.

Residential care, also known as board and care or group home, offers AL services in a smaller environment. These facilities are generally a home converted to suit the needs of a person requiring more assistance. The regulations vary by state; it is important you are familiar with your state's requirements for residential care. Residential care is often less expensive than the other facility options discussed, while providing total care services if needed. Some people like the smaller environment of residential care and find it less intimidating than the larger facilities. These homes generally have the same staff, unlike facilities that may have turnover, which may be difficult for your loved one.

A residential care home provides meals, supportive services such as laundry, activities, personal care, supervision, and limited health-care services. Residential care homes often partner with professionals who can provide additional services if there are health-care needs outside of their ability. Residential care homes can vary greatly. Some rooms are private while others may have two people to a room. Some rooms have a private bathroom or a door to the outside.

If you are considering a facility at some point, there are questions you should ask to determine if your loved one's needs can be met:

- What is the staffing ratio? Is the ratio different at night? What staff is present, such as nursing, nursing assistants, medication techs, and an activity director. For residential care, is there awake staff at night?
- What activities are provided during the day? Ask to see the activity calendar. Visit while activities are occurring to ensure activities are suitable for your loved one and that other residents are engaged. I have been to some facilities that have a calendar, but if residents do not show up, the activity does not occur.
- What safety assurances are in place for a person with dementia? Some facilities have systems where the person with dementia wears a bracelet, known as a wander guard, which prevents them from

wandering off the unit. There are some bracelets that also disable the elevator when the person with dementia is near and a code must be entered to permit the use of the elevator. If this service is not available, is the environment safe for your loved one?

- When was the last Department of Health survey? Ask to see the survey and check for any deficiencies. If there are deficiencies, are they minor and what does the facility do to correct deficiencies?

- What is the cost? Is there one price or additions based on level-of-care needs? Some facilities have one cost no matter the level of care. Many facilities use a tiered approach. The higher the level of care, the higher the cost. For example, if your loved one needs incontinence care, there may be a fee for that. If your loved one is taking many medications or have medications that require an injection, there may be a fee for that as well. Are meals included in the cost? If there are outings, what is your financial obligation?

- How often is the care plan reviewed and updated? How is family included in this process?

- How often is family updated on condition or concerns? What is the process for doing so?

- What services can be provided? What services cannot be provided? If your loved one is already at the maximum capacity of the facility's ability, what will happen if there is a decline?

- Does the facility have the capability to manage behaviors? What occurs if behaviors are not manageable? If a person is transported to acute care for behaviors, can they return to the environment once stable?

I recommend looking at several types of facilities to have a better idea of what the options are. If your loved one can participate, bring him or her along and find out what environment is most desired. Visit at different times of the day, unannounced. Stay for a meal, talk to other residents and their families to understand more about the day-to-day operations.

## Self-Care

Think of ways you have coped with challenging situations in the past. It will be important to maintain the coping strategies that worked in the past to help you through this time. There are some people that turn to maladaptive behaviors when under extreme stress, such as alcohol or drug abuse. If maladaptive behaviors are affecting your everyday life, it is a good time to replace those behaviors with better coping strategies. I know this is easier said than done, but you need to be the best version of yourself to care for a person with dementia. Some people find it useful to engage in counseling therapy. A counselor can listen to your challenges and help you find the best ways to cope. Some people prefer to keep their challenges inside but would benefit from meditation or yoga. Physical activity in general is a great mood enhancer. Getting involved with your local Alzheimer's Association will help you learn more about the disease as well as find resources to help throughout the process. The Alzheimer's Association also has a twenty-four-hour support line where you can speak to someone experienced with dementia care.

# CHAPTER 11:
# AN OFFICER AND HIS BRIDE

One of the hardest things you will ever have to do, my
dear, is to grieve the loss of a person who is still alive.

—Anonymous

Close to Halloween, I received a call from the wellness nurse,
Linda, at a facility I frequented, asking for my assessment of
a married couple in their nineties. Linda stated she is very
concerned about the couple, James and Dorothy Stewart. A
year prior, the Stewarts were living in a casita on the property and moved to IL. Linda, as well as other residents, were
noticing some changes in cognition and questioned their
ability to care for themselves. Additionally, James had a
recent incident that led to the police being called and his
driving privileges were subsequently revoked. Apparently,
James entered his vehicle after concierge drove it to the
front and without noticing a person in front of his vehicle
with a luggage cart, he proceeded to pull forward. The
woman was able to jump out of the way, but the luggage cart
was not so lucky. James did not remember the incident and

continued to drive despite having a revoked license. Linda stated the Stewarts have no living relatives and copies of a POA were not on file.

It was evident on the first meeting the Stewarts suffered from cognitive impairment. Dorothy's cognitive impairment was considerably worse than her husband's. James was short in stature. He stated he was a quarter inch too short of the Navy's standard for manly perfection, yet he was a retired officer in the Navy. He had a couple strands of hair on his head, which he combed to the side. He was soft-spoken and enjoyed joking. His smile and laugh could light up a room. Dorothy had short, white hair and was slightly overweight. She shuffled her feet when she walked and appeared confused through her glasses.

With the extent of cognitive impairment, one of my initial tasks was getting legal affairs in order. Since James was not able to identify anyone who could be responsible legally, I consulted with a fiduciary to initiate a process to ensure the Stewarts would have representation in the event they were not able to make their own decisions. Due to cognitive impairment, we were not sure if a POA would be possible or if the guardianship route would be needed. The IL staff, fortunately, was able to find a family friend from the Stewarts' move-in documents. Their long-time friend, Mark, had known James and Dorothy for most of his life and was willing to serve as a POA. Mark lived about two thousand miles away, but promptly planned a visit to Arizona to get legal documents executed.

In the meantime, I suspected James and Dorothy were neglecting their health-care needs. Neither one could tell me what their health conditions were, who their doctors were, or what medication they were taking. James did indicate they use the Mayo Clinic and was able to bring bottles of medication for himself and his wife for further assessment. James was not aware what the medications were used for or when medication should be taken. It was clear from the date on the prescription bottles and the quantity in the bottles that the medication had not been taken as ordered by their physician. I talked to the Stewarts about getting a mobile physician in to establish care and get their medical needs aligned. Dr. Gray assessed James and Dorothy in their apartment and was able to advise on medications based on the limited medical information we had. James and Dorothy were agreeable to medication boxes being set up and allowing a registered nurse to manage medications. Additionally, a caregiver was initiated for a morning visit to ensure James and Dorothy were taking their medication. After learning Dorothy was taking multiple days of medication in one day, the medication boxes were hidden. Medication compliance was about 90 percent once the system was put in place, which was greatly improved from nearly 0 percent compliance.

Once Mark was in town, he was provided with Life Care Planning documents. The documents were completed, and a mobile notary was able to meet the Stewarts to have the documents signed. Fortunately, they were determined at the time of the signing to have legal capacity. I do believe if we waited any longer, a guardianship would have been the only method for the provision of substituted decision-making.

## GUARDIANSHIP/CONSERVATORSHIP

As you can imagine, when a person with dementia does not have appropriate documents in place and mental capacity is diminished, decision-making will need to go to another competent party. In the absence of a POA, a surrogate decision maker can be appointed. Each state has a hierarchy of health-care surrogates. Examples of a surrogate decision maker is a spouse, adult child, parent, adult sibling, grandparent, or a close friend. In the absence of a surrogate decision maker, a legal proceeding is required to appoint a decision maker. For medical decision-making, a guardian would be appointed, and for financial decision-making and management, a conservator would be appointed. As mentioned previously, this process is lengthy and expensive. A guardianship/conservatorship should be avoided if possible.

There are also situations where family members are available to serve in POA or guardian/conservator roles, but due to misconduct, misappropriation of funds, or feuding within the family, a guardian and/ or conservator is needed to remove or replace family members from decision-making. At times, interested parties choose a method to settle disputes outside of the courtroom by way of an Alternative Dispute Resolution (ADR). This includes mediation and arbitration. Mediation is used to allow interested parties to discuss their feelings, opinions, differences, and concerns with the goal of avoiding a court proceeding by way of negotiating to settle a dispute. Arbitration is a more formal approach and involves an abridged version of a trial, with the goal of coming to an agreement. If parties still have disputes before entering arbitration, they can petition the court to resolve a dispute.

Shortly after meeting James, I placed a lock bar on his steering wheel to deter him from driving because he could not remember he was not supposed to drive. I also disabled his car, to be completely safe. James thought his ability to drive was intact and wanted to see about getting his license back. When I run into situations with clients who believe they can drive, I find it better to go through the steps with them and allow the DMV to make the determination. I transported James to the DMV to determine what his options were. He was told the Medical Review Board revoked his license, and the only way to reinstate his license is to go through the entire process of getting a driver's license (written test, driving test, vision test), in addition to submitting medical records and submitting a statement from his physician stating he is medically safe to drive. The Medical Review Board would review the information and determine if a reinstated license is viable. James walked out of the DMV with his head down and looking completely defeated. He stated he knew he was not going to be able to get his license back and would have to give up driving. Even with cognitive impairment, the event was traumatic enough for him to remember he could no longer drive. James experienced emotional distress over the loss of independence and shame because his wife pushed him to get his driver's license back. I was with him when he broke the news to his wife because he was fearful of her reaction.

The facility staff did a cognitive assessment on James and Dorothy to determine the most appropriate level of care. Based on Dorothy's cognition, it was determined the safest level of care was memory support. James had mild-moderate dementia, while Dorothy had moderate-severe dementia. James and Dorothy wanted to stay together, so the decision was made to move the Stewarts to memory care. The time between meeting James and Dorothy to the time of their move was three months; it all happened quickly.

James and Dorothy were a book-worthy love story. They met as children and married at a young age. James was career military, and they traveled the world. They often spoke of their time in Australia and how those years were the best of their life. They also had a son, who died in his twenties. James was incredibly attentive to his wife and called her his bride. Dorothy's life was James. She was often heard around the apartment screaming for James. James would respond and she would state she did not need anything. It was as though she wanted to make sure he was close by.

Even though their world was turning upside down, they found peace in being together.

I endeavored to allow James and Dorothy as much control over the move as possible. I went through the apartment to figure out what items were necessary in their new environment. We talked about other items that needed to be purchased to make the space their own. I also hired a senior mover, who proved to be especially helpful. On the day of the move, I took James and Dorothy out for lunch. The senior mover had her crew come in, pack up what was going to memory care, and set up the new rooms. Since the memory care was single occupancy, James and Dorothy were in separate rooms. Each room was decorated based on their individual preferences. Once their rooms were ready, I brought the Stewarts to the memory care and showed them to their rooms. They were very confused and wanted to go back to their apartment. We all knew it would be a difficult transition for them.

In the process of the move and immediately after, there were trips to their apartment to get other items that were important to them, as well as the process of setting up services in each room. James was still using a computer, phone, and printer. James and Dorothy also wanted a television in each of their rooms. All the services were transferred and set up so that they had some sense of normalcy.

Because their POA lived across the country, I continued a close working relationship with the Stewarts. This included transferring mail, paying bills, purchasing personal-care supplies, and overall management of their care. James enjoyed having his computer but was forgetting how to use it. I would receive calls at least twice a week indicating he locked himself out of his computer. I had to get an IT expert to help manage his computer use. Since James enjoyed using his computer and it made him feel productive, we kept the computer in his room for quite some time. He also had a telephone, which he did not use on his own, but he felt it was important to have it. I had to buy him a new printer because his current one was very outdated and stopped working. James enjoyed copying coloring pictures and distributing his work around the facility. He had a great sense of pride in that. I was purchasing printer ink frequently, but again, this was important to him, so the expense made sense. I also sold their vehicle and cancelled their automobile insurance.

After a few months in the memory care, I noticed James and Dorothy's cognition start to diminish. Dorothy's dementia was progressing at a much more rapid rate. The challenge was that James and Dorothy's dementia were not as advanced as others on the unit and the decrease in stimulation impacted their minds to a noticeable extent. Dorothy's appetite started to decrease, and since James did not understand what was happening, he would sometimes aggressively encourage her to eat. It got to the point where James and Dorothy had to be separated during meals so that Dorothy could eat in an environment that was less stressful, and in turn, she ate more.

As Dorothy's dementia continued to worsen, James's devoted assistance increased in a non-productive manner. James and Dorothy were separated most of the time. I was not keen on them being separated so much, but the facility stated it was necessary. There were many times James would wander the facility looking for his wife or asking about her. This was a very confusing time for him. In another attempt to care for his wife, James was found in his bathroom washing his wife's panties in his sink. She had an episode of bowel incontinence and he wanted to keep it a secret between the two of them.

James continued to see specialists at the Mayo Clinic, which I accompanied him to. One important appointment we kept up with is the oncologist. James had prostate cancer that was stable, and the oncologist recommended scans at a regular interval to detect any change. In attempt to offer cognitive stimulation I would take James out of the facility to shop and run various errands. I got him set up with the senior center nearby for additional stimulation. I purchased coloring books and jigsaw puzzles for him to keep in his room. Unfortunately, Dorothy was not interested in activities and her abilities to engage in cognitive stimulation were very low.

Dorothy was not used to anyone other than her husband providing care, so the adjustment to memory care proved to be challenging for the staff. Dorothy was very combative with care and did not want anyone to touch her. She was started on medication to help calm her down, as her combativeness was an impediment to receiving even basic care. Management of Dorothy's behaviors was challenging and required multiple interventions. As Dorothy declined, her combativeness started to decrease, although it was present to some extent until her death.

I received a call from the memory-care facility indicating that Dorothy had unintentional, spasmodic movements and that 911 was called. I went to the hospital to be with Dorothy, provide information to the staff, and ensure she was receiving appropriate and compassionate care. The entire experience was confusing and increased her combativeness. After running a battery of tests, the ER physician stated that there is no detectable cause of the movement and that Dorothy was going to be discharged back to the memory-care facility. I, along with three other staff members, helped her to get dressed. She screamed, "Ouch, don't do that!" multiple times. Care was not being provided in an aggressive manner, but Dorothy was so scared and confused she could not cope with the moment.

## EMERGENCY PREPARDNESS

An emergency-room visit is inevitable over the course of the disease. Going to the hospital is a stressful event for anyone, especially for a person with dementia. When a person with dementia is in a different environment, increased confusion occurs. With confusion can also come agitation and even combative behaviors. Obviously, we cannot know when an emergency will occur, but there are actions you can take now to make the situation a little less overwhelming.

Keeping pertinent items together is recommended. Type a document that lists all medications, including over the counter medications, the dosage, and how often the medication is taken. On that document, include allergies to medication, current physicians, and health conditions. You will also want insurance cards readily available. I do recommend having legal paperwork, such as a POA; however, it may get lost in the shuffle, so having a couple of copies may be necessary. I find the less paper, the better.

If your loved one goes to the ER by ambulance, you will want to meet your loved one at the hospital. Typically, once a person arrives to the ER, it takes five-to-ten minutes before the room will open for you to enter. If you bring your loved one to the ER, you will need to be a part of the triage procedure and provide pertinent information. There will be multiple staff members coming into the room, some who are experienced with dementia and others who are not. There will be monitors beeping, X-ray boards maneuvered, and needles poking, as well as various tests. You generally only get a couple of minutes with the ER physician, so you will need to be concise with the information you provide. The nurse will ask for a list of medication; you can provide the document you created and your POA. Staff need to be aware your loved one has dementia, but this should be done in the most respectful manner possible. Your loved one will need you by their side to bring a sense of security and to provide advocacy.

If your loved one is held for observation or admitted to the hospital, you should find out the visiting hours of the hospital and plan to have someone at the bedside at all possible times. A person with dementia may try to pull out IVs, take monitors off, or get out of bed without assistance. A presence will help reinforce the treatment being provided. When I have a client in the hospital, I make it a point to inform the nurse about my client's likes and dislikes and how to handle difficult behaviors. You want the staff to try non-pharmacological methods to manage behaviors instead of turning to medication first, although medication may be needed for safety. Speak to the social worker or discharge planner to start working on a post-hospitalization plan. Ensure you know all your options so that you can make the best decision possible. Some people are transferred to a facility after hospitalization and then back home. The additional change in environment will be confusing, just as it was when going to the hospital.

It is worth mentioning the need to plan for physician appointments. Telling a person with dementia about an appointment days before, or even the night before, usually causes anxiety. I recommend telling your loved one about the appointment about an hour or two before you are going to leave. I have run into situations where a client needs to go to a certain appointment but is resistant to going. In these situations, I do not tell my client we are going to an appointment until the time we leave. When we arrive, I let my client know who we are seeing and why, which gives my client a sense of independence. This is where the medical information document comes in handy. There are many times a physician talks to me and not my client. When this occurs, I ask my client the question the doctor asked and make them a part of the visit. Talking around a person will increase agitation. I had a client who resented going to the doctor because she felt they only talked to me. I would have her hold onto her medication information so she could provide it to the doctor. I also wrote a note saying, "Talk to her. Talking to me causes agitation." This was a very effective method, and my client felt in control of her appointments. After appointments I am generally asked multiple times about what happened in the appointment. I answer the question as if it were the first time I was asked. These moments are about preserving dignity and providing a respectful interaction.

Within several months of the move to memory care, Dorothy was unable to ambulate or transfer without extensive assistance. She was requiring assistance with all her activities of daily living, which included feeding. She was losing weight and sleeping about sixteen hours a day. Six months after Dorothy walked into the memory-care unit, she was placed on hospice services. A DNR was signed by her POA and the decision to focus on quality of life and comfort was made.

Dorothy continued to decline. She spent most of the day sleeping or sitting in a wheelchair staring off into the distance. She ate very little and spoke infrequently. She was eventually bedbound and receiving all care in the bed. James would spend a lot of his day sitting next to her and holding her hand. Because of his cognitive decline he did not understand what was going on. Since James lived day by day or moment by moment, he thought his wife was sick, but did not realize her condition was not reversible. Dorothy died peacefully in the early morning hours, with her husband next to her holding her hand.

## DEMENTIA AND END OF LIFE

While dementia is a progressive, irreversible brain disease, a person does not die from the disease itself. Disease progression and death is the result of the complications of dementia. Some loved ones may choose aggressive treatments to prolong life, while others may choose to allow the disease to take its natural course.

The leading cause of death with dementia is infection. Dementia has debilitating effects, which cause a person with dementia to have a weakened immune system and become more susceptible to infection.

The most common infections are UTIs, respiratory infections, and wound infections. UTIs are common with dementia due to incontinence, inadequate hygiene, and decreased fluid intake. UTIs are treated multiple times through the course of the disease and eventually antibiotics are not effective like they used to be. Even with the best care, UTIs can occur and lead to sepsis. Respiratory infections are also common, but most commonly is aspiration pneumonia. As a person with dementia declines, the ability to swallow is impaired, causing food and fluids to enter the lungs. Aspiration does not always cause pneumonia, but the risk is high. If a person with dementia is coughing when eating or drinking, dietary changes may be needed. A person with dementia should never be forced to eat. Some loved ones may choose to have a feeding tube placed for artificial nutrition due to weight loss; however, there is still a risk of aspiration and pneumonia.

Lastly, wounds can occur with end-stage dementia due to immobility. Skin breakdown can progress rapidly and require skilled intervention. Wounds are highly susceptible to infection and are difficult to heal once they progress. Additionally, decreased nutritional intake impacts the ability to heal. Once a person with dementia is bedbound, special attention needs to be paid to the skin, keeping it clean and dry and turning every two hours. Again, even with great care, wounds can develop.

Falls are common with dementia, but falls with injury can accelerate the disease process. I am sure you have heard a story about an elderly person falling, breaking their hip, and dying from pneumonia soon after. When an injury from a fall occurs, the person with dementia may require surgery and less mobility may result. It is also more difficult to come out of anesthesia when dementia is present. Physical therapy to assist with mobility is less effective with dementia due to difficulty understanding prompts, slowed cognitive function, and difficulty following a consistent program. With immobility comes all the potential complications as mentioned in the last paragraph. Additionally, if a person on a blood thinner falls, they are at a high risk of bleeding or internal hemorrhage, which can be a medical emergency. Fractures are not necessarily caused by a fall. With advanced age and decreased bone mass, spontaneous fractures can occur. These are hard to detect because there is no precipitating event. Anytime acute pain is present, a fracture should be ruled out.

Embolus, also known as blood clots, are also a complication of being immobile. There are people who wear compression stockings when flying to avoid blood clots, so we know there is potential for them to occur rapidly. Blood clots can travel, leading to complications such as heart attack and stroke. Blood clots can also travel to the lungs, known as a pulmonary embolus, and can present with acute difficulty breathing.

Let us not forget, a person with dementia can also have other disease processes. These conditions can also be a cause of death. For example, a person with dementia can also have extensive heart disease and suffer heart failure. Dementia may confound any co-morbid illnesses and cause the person to be more susceptible from complications from another disease process.

The death of a spouse is a traumatic event for anyone, but the death of a spouse when impaired cognition is present brings about other aspects of suffering. James's short-term memory was impaired to the extent that he did not remember his wife had passed. Every morning he would go to her room and found an empty bed. He would look around the memory-care unit for her and ask staff where his wife was. He would learn of his wife's death and experienced the trauma of hearing that news multiple times a day. At times, the staff would tell him a therapeutic fib and redirect him to spare him the shock. When I would visit, he would tell me they took his wife away. He knew his wife was not there, but in his mind he could not explain it. The only logical explanation in his mind was she was taken away. Our conversations were difficult. I wanted to make sure I understood the feeling behind his statements and enter his reality, instead of forcing him into my reality. In time, he seemed to know his wife died and appeared to be coping well.

James's ability to ambulate became progressively worse, and it was no longer safe to take him out of the memory care without wheelchair assistance. To increase stimulation, a caregiver was brought in to spend time doing activities with him. They would put together jigsaw puzzles and color pictures. James enjoyed the personal one-on-one attention. As dementia goes, James continued to decline. Once James was no longer able to ambulate, I requested a hospice evaluation. James was considered eligible for hospice services. A DNR order for James had been initiated at the time his wife's DNR was completed. The decline James experienced was much slower than his wife.

As mentioned, James was career military, serving thirty years in the Navy. He retired as a captain and was very proud of his service. Before he moved to memory care, I found short stories he wrote for a writing group he was a part of. I kept the stories and provided a copy to him. When I meet a client for the first time, I only know information that is pertinent to the care they need. Over time I get to know more about them; I felt James's stories provided even more insight into his life. At fourteen years old his father told him to stop playing with toy airplanes and go out into the cold world and get a job. He joined the Civil Air Patrol in the middle of World War II. At that time, he was making twenty-five dollars a week, which was more than some of the adult men were making. Just days after his eighteenth birthday, he applied for entrance into the Navy's pilot training program. His first assignment out of school was in French Morocco where he flew Hellcat fighter planes. One story, titled *Tsingtao*, was about his time on an aircraft carrier during World War II. He was tasked to fly over Nationalist China with cameras on their Hellcat fighters to make photo mosaic maps. He talked about the archaic technology of that time and the difficulty in knowing where to go. He had other stories of near attacks that seem to be secrets that very few know about. When James did retire, he and Dorothy moved to San Juan Island where he rebuilt a World War I airplane that is now showcased in a Seattle museum. James often thought he was on a Navy ship and asked why he was on the bottom of the ship and wanted to know how to be upgraded. Interestingly enough, he was on the bottom level in the memory-care facility. As he declined, his memories were back to his Navy days, where his bride was young, and he was waiting for the next important mission.

The National Hospice and Palliative Care Organization in collaboration with the Department of Veterans Affairs has a program called We Honor Veterans. Under this program, a hospice organization provides educational tools and resources to help hospice staff understand the unique needs of a veteran and to improve quality of care for veterans. Some veterans choose to have a pinning ceremony where they are honored for their service and are given the opportunity to tell their story. The hospice caring for James did a ceremony for him. His caregiver and many of the staff at the facility were there. I was running a little behind. When I arrived, the ceremony had started, but James stopped midsentence, pointed at me and gave a big smile. James did not really know who I was to him but did tell me I was the person that helps him. The smile he gave me that day made my day.

Until COVID-19, he enjoyed visits from myself and the caregiver. Once the pandemic started, visits from myself and the caregiver were stopped. The only visitor James was allowed was the hospice nurse every fourteen days. Although his cognitive decline continued, other aspects evaluated by hospice that indicate overall decline were not present. James did not have any wounds; he was not getting infections and his weight was stable. During the pandemic, James was taken off hospice for an extended prognosis.

James was doing well in the memory-care facility, until December when I was notified he was positive for COVID-19. In addition, he was found to have bronchitis. He was treated for the bronchitis and quarantined to his room for COVID-19. He amazingly pulled through this and turned ninety-six the following month. Unfortunately, the staff noticed blood in his urine, and eventually he experienced urinary retention. A catheter was placed, and James was admitted onto hospice services again, with a terminal diagnosis of prostate cancer.

After COVID-19 vaccines were provided to residents and infection rates decreased, senior facilities began to open to visitors, although there were rules to optimize safety. I set up an appointment to visit with James. As I walked toward the common area in the memory-care unit, I saw a man in a wheelchair and had to ask the staff if James was in the wheelchair. He was barely recognizable to me. The staff brought him to his room so that we could visit.

James appeared thin and frail. He was unable to hold himself up in the wheelchair and required foot pedals to avoid slipping out of the chair. He was wearing a hat, but I could see hair growth around the edge of the hat. I did not realize he could grow hair on the sides of his head. As I suspected, James did not recognize me. I talked to him briefly but could recognize his verbal skills were greatly reduced. He could put some words together, but some of his sentences contained words that should not go together. I wheeled him to the table in his room and tried to put a small puzzle together with him. He was no longer able to participate. Since the puzzle was small, I was able to put it together quickly and talk to him about what he could see in the picture. Afterward, I read one of his short stories out loud. I had hoped to spark old memories. He commented, "I wish I could remember that." His greatest joy at this point in his disease was sitting with another person and knowing he was not alone.

I have witnessed the effect of a pandemic on the elderly community and especially those with dementia. Although dementia is a progressive disease, the decline has been much more rapid. Despite efforts to promote normalcy, the pandemic has amplified the negative influence of social isolation. Many of my clients have expressed feeling like they are in prison and suffer a complete loss of independence. If anything, this pandemic has solidified my belief that the elderly thrive from social interaction; just being present means the world.

# CHAPTER 12:
# FINDING HUMOR AND JOY

He who laughs, lasts.

—Norwegian Proverb

Although the dementia journey can be stressful and feel impossible at times, there are moments that bring your devotion into perspective. I hope you have experienced these moments and have found the joy in caring for a person with dementia. If we can learn to live in the moment without expectations and be truly present, we may find pleasure in the unique relationship we can share with a person with dementia. There may be tender moments, or silly moments, or even tears that turn into laughter. I want to conclude this book by telling short stories about some moments I have had while caring for many precious people living with dementia.

One of my favorite clients was residing in an IL apartment and was needing significant help. She stated she will not move to the care center, so twenty-four-hour home care was initiated. She was an absolute sweetheart. I met her when she was ninety-nine years old. She enjoyed dressing up and putting on makeup when going to the dining room. One day the caregiver was putting mascara on her and she commented, "Don't put too much, the other women will get jealous," followed by a laugh. Her children would visit often, and I could tell by the interactions my client was an incredible mother. Her daughter was telling her a story and her responses were so tender and heartfelt. I commented on how sweet she was. My client turned to look at me and said, "Oh, I can get a lot sweeter." I believed every word of it. When she turned one hundred, I went to the facility to find her sitting in her electric wheelchair, looking gorgeous as always. She put her arms in the air and said, "I'm one hundred!"

I cared for a client who was a retired nurse practitioner. I was told by family she was also a stand-up comedian. She would walk around her apartment singing made up songs while moving her arms as though she was flying. We were getting ready to go out one day and she asked me to get a wheelchair, as she was having pain that day. She told me not to get the wicker wheelchair because she did not like it. She was joking of course. I grabbed a wheelchair and came back, stating I could only find the whicker wheelchair. She looked at me confused and asked, "What are you talking about?" having no recollection of her comment moments before. I laughed, saying, "I don't know; I'm just crazy today." She laughed and continued singing. There was another time where we had a psychologist do an examination on her due to cognitive decline. I was present for a part of it, which she did not remember after the fact. The story she told her family of that visit was of a sweaty man who showed up and looked like he was going to pass out. She invited him in, gave him water, and tried to help him feel better. She said he was there for five minutes, asked about animals, then left. She talked about the sweaty man for about two years after the fact. Each time she told the story, she added a little more information. The visit with the psychologist was not at all what she described, but that was the story in her mind. When she told the story, I could not help but to smile and laugh along with her. Unfortunately, she contracted COVID-19 and died very rapidly afterward.

Since my business also includes the in-home care piece, I find myself filling in for shifts as needed. We had a darling client, whose husband was a high school teacher and needed someone during the day while he was at work. He was very devoted to his wife and wanted her to remain at home for as long as possible. She loved watching *I Love Lucy* and would watch old episodes throughout the day. One day we watched the famous scene of Lucy and Ethel at the chocolate factory, where they could not keep up with the production line. In a frenzy, Lucy and Ethel began to eat the chocolates, stuffing their mouths full before reverting to putting chocolates in their hats and in their clothing. My client laughed and said, "Oh, Lucy," in the sweetest voice, followed by a giggle. Every episode when Lucy did something silly, she had the same reaction. At one point, I was using the restroom and heard her say, "Oh, Lucy," and she giggled. I giggled in the bathroom after hearing her. I enjoyed watching *I Love Lucy* with her just to listen to her reaction.

My staff and I were called in to help a woman with dementia with behaviors in the assisted living facility where she resided. She would vacillate between charming and irrational behavior, without any warning. I received a call one day indicating she asked the caregiver if she could borrow their phone. Once she received the phone, she ran to the elevator, got in, and got the door closed before the caregiver could get to her. The staff at the facility had to check all the floors to find her. In one of her charming moments, she told my caregiver she could help her with her high forehead. She got out a brush and showed her how to brush her forehead to make hair grow in. My caregiver called me in tears from laughter. I can only imagine being there in that moment.

A client with middle-stage dementia was still living home alone with minimal caregiver support. I received a call from the caregiver indicating the client was not home. She was still driving at that time, so there was no telling where she went. Minutes later, the client came walking down the street with grocery bags. Once in the house, the caregiver asked the client where her car was. The client had no idea. Come to find out, the client drove to the store, forgot she drove, and walked back. The caregiver drove her to the store to get her car and followed her back home. She did not have a vehicle much longer after that incident. The client had a carefree attitude, and I never saw her rattled. In fact, I would attend her neurology appointments, and when the neurologist would ask her the date to assess her orientation, she would state, "I don't know, and I don't care." She would throw her arms up and state it does not matter. She answered almost every question in this manner. I would say she was pleasantly confused.

I cared for a man who had dementia related to traumatic brain injuries. He enjoyed telling jokes and making people laugh. He also had a bit of a drinking problem. One day he came home from a night of heavy drinking and the caregiver was at the home waiting for him. He lived in a two-story condo and upon arriving home, he attempted to throw his cane up the stairs. The cane came down the stairs, so he tried again. The caregiver told me he tried a handful of times before allowing her to take his cane upstairs. There was an area at the bottom on the stairs that was a circular shape and indented to the point where there was nearly a hole. I asked him about the area, and he stated he did not know what happened. After hearing the cane story, I became almost positive he was falling down the stairs and crashing into the wall. Due to his head injury, he tried to memorize various dates, jokes, and stories to preserve cognition. He asked me if I ever heard of the nonconforming sparrow. I had not. He then told me he met a foreign-government top official who was known to be very serious. He told the story of the nonconforming sparrow and got a slight smile. I do not know who wrote the story, but here it is:

## If You Are Unhappy

Once upon a time, there was a nonconforming sparrow
who decided not to fly south for the winter.
However, soon the weather turned so cold he reluctantly
started to fly south.
In a short time, ice began to form on his wings. Almost
frozen, he fell to earth, landing in a barnyard.
A cow passed by and crapped on the little sparrow and the
sparrow thought it was the end.
But the manure warmed him and defrosted his wings.
Warm and happy and able to breathe he started to sing.
Just then a large cat came by and hearing the chirping,
investigated the sound.
The cat cleared away the manure, found the chirping bird
and promptly ate him.
The moral of the story is:
Everyone who s**ts on you is not necessarily your enemy.
Everyone who gets you out of the s**t is not necessarily
your friend.
If you're warm and happy in a pile of s**t, keep your
mouth shut.

One of the most beautiful stories I have watched was of
Naomi Feil integrating music into a therapy session to
enhance communication with her patient, Gladys Wilson. I
was introduced to this video early in my dementia learning
journey, but the affect was so insightful that I will never
forget it. Naomi sings a familiar song to Gladys, who was
living with Alzheimer's disease and was essentially non-
verbal. Eventually Gladys begins to tap her hand to the beat

of the song, and while Naomi was mirroring her intensity to Gladys, Gladys began to sign along.

## THE POWER OF MUSIC

Music has a profound effect on people with dementia. I use music when a client is agitated and when I am trying to introduce stimulation. I have a client with intense behavioral disturbances and have found music is one of the only ways to decrease his agitation. He can go from calling me every name in the book to being pleasant and playful. I dance a little and then he dances, and it is almost as though he is a different person.

I was with a client at a memory-care facility recently and the staff was playing familiar music with the words to the songs running across the television. Residents match the intensity of the music, so a slow song will calm and a fast song will excite them. When the faster music was on, they got up and danced and had a great time. Slow music is also important with dementia, as it does promote a calm atmosphere. I always thought slow, calm music would ease an agitated client, but learned from a music therapist this not the case. The music therapist stated music should match the intensity of the client and then can be scaled down to calmer music to help calm their mood. If a client is screaming, music can be loud and more rapid and then the sound and intensity can decrease over a period.

I hope this book has supported your efforts to learn about dementia and how to provide optimal care. I hope this book has also provided reassurance in your abilities to care for a person with dementia and the strength to know you are not alone in this journey. This journey may be the most diffi- cult experience in your life and will be imperfect, but you are perfectly capable. Never forget to take care of yourself!

# Resources

AARP (Assessing Driving Ability):
www.aarp.org/auto/driver-safety/driving-assessment.

Advanced Directives: www.nhpco.org/advancedirective.

Aging Life Care Expert (Care Manager) locator:
www.aginglifecare.org.

Alzheimer's Association: www.alz.org.

Alzheimer's Association 24-hour help line: 1-800-272-3900.

Alzheimer's Store: www.alzstore.com.

CarFit: www.car-fit.org.

Caring Bridge (Stay connected with friends and family):
www.caringbridge.org.

Centers for Medicare and Medicare & Medicaid Services:
www.cms.gov.

Extra Help Program (Medication Assistance): 1-800-772-1213
or www.socialsecurity.gov/prescriptionhelp.

Federal Trade Commission (Do Not Call Registry):
www.donotcall.gov.

HUD Exchange (Counseling): www.hudexchange.info/programs/housing-counseling.

Long Term Services & Supports for Medicaid: www.medicaid.gov/medicaid/long-term-services-supports/index.html.

Lotsa Helping Hands (Organize care): www.lotsahelpinghands.com.

Mediator Locator: www.mediate.com/mediator/search.cfm.

Medicare & You: www.cms.gov/Outreach-and-Education/Outreach/Partnerships/MY.

Medicare Compare: www.medicare.gov/care-compare.

National Academy of Elder Law Attorneys: www.naela.org.

National Hospice and Palliative Care Organization: www.nhpco.org.

Paying for Senior Care: www.payingforseniorcare.com.

Senior Care Management Solutions, LLC: www.scms.com.

Social Security Administration: 1-800-772-1213 or www.ssa.gov.

True Link card: www.truelinkfinancial.com.

VA Pension Benefits: www.va.gov/pension.

# Bibliography

## Chapter 1:
## What Is Dementia?

Alzheimer's Association. "Types of Dementia." What Is
Dementia? Accessed March 27, 2020.
https://www.alz.org/alzheimers-dementia/what-is-
dementia/types-of-dementia.

Heintz, Hannah, Patrick Monette, Gary Epstein-Lubow, Lorie
Smith, Susan Rowlett, and Brent P. Forester.
"Emerging Collaborative Care Models for Dementia
Care in the Primary Care Setting: A Narrative Review."
*The American Journal of Geriatric Psychiatry* 28, no. 3
(2020): 320–30.

Lewy Body Dementia Association. *Diagnosing and Managing
Lewy Body Dementia: A Comprehensive Guide for
Healthcare Professionals*. Atlanta, GA: LBDA, 2017.
https://www.lbda.org/wp-content
uploads/2020/09/3737-lbda-physicians-book-
22dec17.pdf.

Mayo Clinic. "Frontotemporal dementia." Diseases &
Conditions. Last Modified January 8, 2021.

https://www.mayoclinic.org/diseases-conditions/frontotemporal-dementia/symptoms-causes/syc-20354737.

Reisberg, Barry, Steven Ferris, Mony de Leon, and Thomas Crook. "The Global Deterioration Scale for Assessment of Primary Degenerative Dementia." *American Journal of Psychiatry* 139, no. 9 (1982): 1136–39.

## Chapter 2:
## I Think My Mom Has Dementia

Reisberg, Barry. "Functional assessment staging (FAST)." *Psychopharmacol Bull* 24, no. 4 (1988): 653–9.

## Chapter 3:
## A Dementia Diagnosis Alone Is Not Enough

Ballard, C., J. Waite, (2002). "The effectiveness of atypical antipsychotics for the treatment of agitation and psychosis in Alzheimer's disease." *Cochrane Database of Systematic Reviews* 1 (January 2006).

Cook, Joan, Elissa McCarthy, and Steven Thorp. "Older adults with PTSD: Brief State of Research and Evidence-Based Psychotherapy Case Illustration." *The American Journal of Geriatric Psychiatry* 25, no. 5 (2017): 522–30.

Sjöberg, Linnea, Laura Fratiglioni, Martin Lövdén, and Hui-Xin Wang. "Low Mood and Risk of Dementia: The Role of Marital Status and Living Situation." *The American Journal of Geriatric Psychiatry* 28, no. 1 (2020): 33–44.

## Chapter 4:
## Managing Behaviors

Alzheimer's Association. "Wandering." Stages and Behaviors. Accessed May 10, 2020. https://www.alz.org/help-support/caregiving/stages-behaviors/wandering.

Davis, Daniel, Donal Skelly, Carol Murray, Edel Hennessy, Jordan Bowen, Samuel Norton, Carol Brayne, Terhi Rakkonen, Raimo Sulkava, David Sanderson, Nicholas Rawlins, David Bannerman, Alasdair MacLullich, and Colm Cunningham. "Worsening Cognitive Impairment and Neurodegenerative Pathology Progressively Increase Risk for Delirium." *The American Journal of Geriatric Psychiatry* 23, no. 4 (2015): 403–15.

Müller-Spahn, F. "Behavioral Disturbances in Dementia." *Dialogues in Clinical Neuroscience* 5, no. 1 (2003): 49–59.

Reisberg, Barry. "Functional assessment staging (FAST)." *Psychopharmacol Bull* 24, no. 4 (1988): 653–9.

Reisberg, Barry, Emile Franssen, Liduin Souren, Stefanie Auer, Imran Akram, and Sunnie Kenowsky. "Evidence and Mechanisms of Retrogenesis in Alzheimer's and Other Dementias: Management and Treatment

Import." *American Journal of Alzheimer's Disease & Other Dementias* 17, no. 4 (2002): 202–12.

## Chapter 5:
## Supported Self-Destruction

Chee, Justin, Carol Hawley, Judith Charlton, Shawn Marshall, Ian Gillespie, Sjaan Koppel, Brenda Vrkljan, Debbie Ayotte, and Mark Rapoport. "Risk of Motor Vehicle Collision or Driving Impairment after Traumatic Brain Injury: A Collaborative International Systematic Review and Meta-Analysis." *Journal of Head Trauma Rehabilitation* 34, no. 1 (2019): 27–38.

## Chapter 6:
## Where You Going with Those?

"Fitness-to-Drive screening measure online." Accessed March 13, 2021. http://fitnesstodrive.phhp.ufl.edu/.

CarFit, "Order Form." Downloads. Accessed March 13, 2021. https://www.car-fit.org/downloads/CarFitPromoOrderForm-2015.pdf.

Chee, Justin, Carol Hawley, Judith Charlton, Shawn Marshall, Ian Gillespie, Sjaan Koppel, Brenda Vrkljan, Debbie Ayotte, and Mark Rapoport. "Risk of Motor Vehicle Collision or Driving Impairment after Traumatic Brain Injury: A Collaborative International Systematic Review and Meta-Analysis." *Journal of Head Trauma Rehabilitation* 34, no.1 (2019): 27–38.

## Chapter 7:
## Resources to Provide Care

"What's Medicare?" Your Medicare coverage choices. Accessed February 1, 2021.
https://www.medicare.gov/what-medicare-covers/
your-medicare-coverage-choices/whats-medicare.

Centers for Medicare & Medicaid Services. "FFS & MA NOMNC/DENC." Beneficiary Notices Initiative (BNI). Accessed January 11, 2021.
https://www.cms.gov/Medicare/Medicare-General-
Information/BNI/FFS-Expedited-Determination-
Notices.

IRS. "Credit for the Elderly or the Disabled at a Glance." Credits & Deductions. Accessed January 25, 2021.
https://www.irs.gov/credits-deductions/individuals/
credit-for-the-elderly-or-the-disabled.

Paying for Senior Care. "Federal Tax Credit for Elderly Dependent Care." Accessed January 25, 2021.
https://www.payingforseniorcare.com/caregivers/
dependent_care_tax_credit.

Paying for Senior Care. "Free Assistance Finding Quality, Affordable, Elder Care." Accessed January 25, 2021.

https://www.payingforseniorcare.com/home-care-assisted-living/find-affordable-elder-care.

Paying for Senior Care. "Long Term Care Insurance and Paying for Elder Care." Accessed January 25, 2021. https://www.payingforseniorcare.com/financial-products/insurance/ltc_insurance.

Paying for Senior Care. "Pay for Aging Care by Converting a Life Insurance Policy." Accessed January 25, 2021. https://www.payingforseniorcare.com/lifecare-assurance-benefit-plan.

Paying for Senior Care. "Using Reverse Mortgages to Pay for Long Term Care." Accessed January 25, 2021. https://www.payingforseniorcare.com/financial-products/reverse-mortgages.

Social Security Administration. "What Is Supplemental Security Income?" SSI Home Page. Accessed February 1, 2021. https://www.ssa.gov/ssi/.

Society of Certified Senior Advisors. *Financial and Estate Planning for Age 65 and Older: A Professional's Guide to Contemporary Issues of Aging.* Society of Certified Senior Advisors, 2015.

Veterans Affairs. "Eligibility for Veteran's Pension." Eligibility. Accessed February 1, 2021. https://www.va.gov/pension/eligibility/.

Veterans Affairs. "VA health care." Health Care. Accessed February 1, 2021. https://www.va.gov/health-care/.

Veterans Affairs. "VA pension benefits." Pension. Accessed February 1, 2021. https://www.va.gov/pension/.

## Chapter 8:
## Till Death Do Us Part

American Stroke Association. "Types of Stroke." About Stroke. Accessed November 16, 2020. https://www.stroke.org/en/about-stroke/types-of-stroke.

Arizona Attorney General. "Consumer Scams." Seniors. Accessed August 23, 2020. https://www.azag.gov/seniors/consumer-scams.

FBI. "Elder Fraud." Common Scams and Crimes. Accessed August 23, 2020. https://www.fbi.gov/scams-and-safety/common-scams-and-crimes/elder-fraud.

World Population Review. "Gun ownership by country 2021." Country Rankings. Accessed March 22, 2021. https://worldpopulationreview.com/country-rankings/gun-ownership-by-country.

## Chapter 9:
## A New Beginning

Alzheimer's Association. "Home Safety Checklist." Resources.
    https://www.alz.org/help-support/resources/home_
    safety_checklist.

Alzheimer's Association. "Korsakoff syndrome." Types of
    Dementia. Accessed December 12, 2020.
    https://www.alz.org/alzheimers-dementia/what-is-
    dementia/types-of-dementia/korsakoff-syndrome.

## Chapter 10:
## Taking Care of You

Alzheimer's Association. "Residential Care." Care Options.
    Accessed June 7, 2021.
    https://www.alz.org/help-support/caregiving/care-
    options/residential-care.

## Chapter 11:
## An Officer and His Bride

Cornell Law School. "Alternative Dispute Resolution." Wex.
    Accessed March 29, 2021.
    https://www.law.cornell.edu/wex/alternative_
    dispute_resolution.

## Chapter 12:
## Finding Humor and Joy

Memorybridge. "Gladys Wilson and Naomi Feil." YouTube,
    video uploaded in 2009.
        https://www.youtube.com/watch?v=CrZXz10FcVM.

# About the Author

Melissa Johnson completed a bachelor's in the science of nursing from Arizona State University in 2005 and has dedicated her nursing career to caring for the elderly. Melissa also obtained a master's in health care administration from University of Phoenix in 2009. Melissa holds a certification in hospice and palliative nursing, as she believes end-of-life care is just as important as obtaining a dementia diagnosis, managing the challenges dementia presents, and guiding loved ones through the process. Prior to establishing Senior Care Management Solutions, LLC with her husband, Ryan Johnson, Melissa obtained a certification in case management. She has volunteered for the Alzheimer's Association since 2011, providing community education about Alzheimer's disease and related dementias. Melissa wrote this book because she believes it is important to use her knowledge to help others through their journey.